T0348910

Acclaim for *What Happened to My Sex Life?*

"*What Happened to My Sex Life?* is for anyone who has ever felt disconnected, overwhelmed, or frustrated by their fluctuating sexual desire. Dr. Balestrieri's book will help you identify what's getting in the way of your desire and give you tools to move toward the sex life you deserve. Let this book be a guide back to yourself, your body, your desire, and your pleasure."**—Emily Morse, author of** *Smart Sex* **and host of the** *Sex with Emily* **podcast**

"Dr. Kate Balestrieri brilliantly explores and normalizes all of the very real and very understandable reasons we end up feeling detached from our sex lives. And she provides us with steps we can take to proudly reconnect to our sexuality. Here's to shedding shame and reclaiming pleasure!"**—Alexandra H. Solomon, PhD, author of** *Love Every Day* **and** *Loving Bravely* **and host of the** *Reimagining Love* **podcast**

"If you've lost your desire and are struggling to feel pleasure and connection, this book is for you. Written with compassion and full of stories of real people, it is an invaluable resource for anyone who wants to know where their sex drive went—and importantly, how to get it back."**—Laurie Mintz, PhD, author of** *A Tired Woman's Guide to Passionate Sex* **and** *Becoming Cliterate*

"As someone deeply invested in understanding the complexities of human desire and relationships, I found this book to be an enlightening and essential read. Dr. Balestrieri masterfully navigates the intricate landscape of desire, addressing both internal and interpersonal factors that can lead to a loss of libido. Her compassionate approach reassures readers that they are not alone or broken, but rather on a journey to rediscover their authentic desires. This book is a valuable resource for anyone seeking to understand and rekindle their sexual vitality. I highly recommend it to anyone looking to deepen their connection with themselves and their partners."**—Shan Boodram, certified sex educator and author of** *The Game of Desire*

"This truly brilliant book is a must-read for any woman having trouble accessing sexual pleasure. It encourages exploration of all the factors—personal, relational, political, and cultural—that impact our sexual selves, and offers evidence-based information, thought-provoking questions, case studies, and suggestions to help promote sexual and relational wellness. It educates, inspires, and guides, taking the reader on an incredible journey of self-discovery and empowerment. Bravo!"
—Nan Wise, PhD, certified sex therapist, sex neuroscience researcher, and author of *Why Good Sex Matters*

"Balestrieri explores the various roots of sexual stagnation, grants permission to have pleasure, safety, anger, and boundaries, and provides actionable steps for reconnecting with one's body. Balestrieri's multidisciplinary approach to reconnecting with sexual pleasure is relatable for anyone struggling with their sex life, no matter where they are on their journey. Her book is a must-read for those seeking to better understand themselves and their relationship with sexual pleasure."
—Zachary Zane, sex columnist and author of *Boyslut: A Memoir and Manifesto*

"*What Happened to My Sex Life?* is the smart, deeply vulnerable, and empowering guide people are craving. Dr. Balestrieri offers an insightful lens on barriers to desire and, most importantly, innovative strategies for finding our way back to the sex lives we deserve."**—Dr. Holly Richmond,** author of *Reclaiming Pleasure*

"*What Happened to My Sex Life?* is an invaluable guide for anyone struggling with low sexual desire or feeling disconnected from their sexuality. Dr. Balestrieri offers compassionate insights and practical advice to help readers address the many factors that can lead to a loss of connection with their sexual selves."**—Sarah E. Hill,** author of *This Is Your Brain on Birth Control*

"This indispensable guide deserves a place on every bedside table, whether you're in a relationship or not. Balestrieri deftly decodes our seemingly insurmountable hang-ups around sex and intimacy to prove that we're not alone, we're not abnormal, and we're not without tools to regain our own personal connection to desire."**—Ali Drucker,** author of *Do As I Say, Not Who I Did*

What Happened to My Sex Life?

What Happened to My Sex Life?

A Sex Therapist's Guide to Reclaiming Lost Desire, Connection and Pleasure

Dr. Kate Balestrieri

THE EXPERIMENT

NEW YORK

The Experiment, LLC
220 East 23rd Street, Suite 600
New York, NY 10010-4658
theexperimentpublishing.com

This book contains the opinions and ideas of its author. It is intended to provide helpful and informative material on the subjects addressed in the book. It is sold with the understanding that the author and publisher are not engaged in rendering medical, health, or any other kind of personal professional services in the book. The author and publisher specifically disclaim all responsibility for any liability, loss, or risk—personal or otherwise—that is incurred as a consequence, directly or indirectly, of the use and application of any of the contents of this book.

THE EXPERIMENT and its colophon are registered trademarks of The Experiment, LLC. Many of the designations used by manufacturers and sellers to distinguish their products are claimed as trademarks. Where those designations appear in this book and The Experiment was aware of a trademark claim, the designations have been capitalized.

The Experiment's books are available at special discounts when purchased in bulk for premiums and sales promotions as well as for fund-raising or educational use. For details, contact us at info@theexperimentpublishing.com.

Library of Congress Cataloging-in-Publication Data

Names: Balestrieri, Kate, author.
Title: What happened to my sex life? : a sex therapist's guide to reclaiming lost desire, connection, and pleasure / Dr. Kate Balestrieri.
Description: New York : The Experiment, [2025] | Includes bibliographical references and index.
Identifiers: LCCN 2024046761 (print) | LCCN 2024046762 (ebook) | ISBN 9781891011764 (hardcover) | ISBN 9781891011771 (ebook)
Subjects: LCSH: Sex instruction. | Sexual excitement. | Sexual disorders.
Classification: LCC HQ31 .B2398 2025 (print) | LCC HQ31 (ebook) | DDC 613.9--dc23/eng/20241118
LC record available at https://lccn.loc.gov/2024046761
LC ebook record available at https://lccn.loc.gov/2024046762

ISBN 978-1-891011-76-4
Ebook ISBN 978-1-891011-77-1

Jacket and text design by Beth Bugler
Author photograph courtesy of the author

Manufactured in the United States of America

First printing February 2025
10 9 8 7 6 5 4 3 2 1

To every woman who has felt disconnected from herself, from pleasure, from sensuality, or at odds with desire at some point in her life: You are not alone, and you deserve a relationship with sex that is self-defined, empowered, and full of pleasure.

I hope you find some solace within the pages of this book and a path back to yourself.

Contents

Introduction

"Bu t you're a sex therapist!" my good friend Betty shrieked. Having known me for almost twenty years, she was gob-smacked to learn that my partner and I had had sex only once that entire year. To be honest, so was I. I hadn't really said it out loud to anyone but my own therapist, and it felt like such a stark divergence with who I am, not only as a sex therapist, but as a person. I love sex! I love the study of it, the sounds, the smell, the feel, and of course . . . the pleasure!

Betty knew me through and through and after the heckling stopped, she quietly asked, "What's going on?" I swirled my glass of Nebbiolo, took a sip, and tried to count the notes of tannin to buy a little time in my response. The truth was I'd lost my connection to sex over time *and* all at once. It happened because of everything and nothing. There was no one thing to point at because there were many seemingly small or insignificant reasons. Somehow, sex just became less important to me, surely that had to be the case? Maybe I spent too much time talking and thinking about sex, and disinterest in having it was a casualty of my work. Maybe I was starting peri-menopause? Maybe my partner and I weren't right anymore? Maybe it was because I'd gained some weight? Or was the weight a side effect of something else? Maybe I was bored?

Except I wasn't bored or disinterested: I felt completely disconnected from my sexuality and from my libido. It was as if sex were an old friend and we'd fallen out of contact, only to barely recognize each other anymore. I missed it, thought of it fondly, wondered what it would feel like to be connected again, but hadn't prioritized it. My sexuality felt so separate from me, I wondered if I was ever going to have sex again. Solo or partnered, sex in my personal life just stopped occurring to me.

Betty was having none of my stall tactics and jumped in with several hypotheses. "Are you and [my partner] doing okay? You're working too much! How's your health?" I took another sip of wine and my eyes got a little teary. It was hard to have this discussion, because doing so made it real. Who was I? Was I even myself anymore?

The last time my partner and I were intimate was already six months previously. Before that, it had been ten months. We were stuck. Dead in the water, except there was no water—just a pile of dry earth. It had been so long, it was awkward. We didn't know what to do at first or how to even get started. It's not like we hadn't discussed our once-hot-now-languishing sex life, but neither of us knew how to reclaim it. We were both feeling confused, resentful, and rejected. It was a conversation we had regularly, and while there was no one to blame, there didn't seem to be a satisfactory answer or solution. We both kept on powering through the day-to-day of our sexless lives.

We were completely out of rhythm, out of sync. Though there were moments when our bodies felt familiar, we were like actors replaying an old script—we had all the right props, but so much had happened in our lives since the last time we were together, it seemed the lines no longer made sense. Those characters had grown stale, and although they were roles we once relished, they now felt flat and uninspired. When we did it, I was relieved that we'd *had* sex and finally interrupted our streak of unintentional abstinence, yet I still didn't feel like me.

Dessert arrived: a pistachio molten lava cake. We were at one of my favorite Italian restaurants and this was my guilty pleasure, but in that moment, it fell flat. The cake looked the same and tasted the same—it had the perfect cake to lava ratio and a pistachio flavor that was not too sweet. Betty, whose patience for my answer had run out, started eyeballing my picked-over dessert. "Are you going to finish that?" she probed with a hopeful smirk. "No, take it," I said even though the cake was as delicious as I recalled. *It was me who was flat.* I took another sip of wine while I tried to piece together what had been running through my mind in the last few minutes. "I don't know how to answer you about my sex life," I blurted out, "I feel completely detached from it."

Betty finished my cake and jokingly chided that she did not feel disconnected from her sexuality, so I should pass along some of those free sex toys that various brands send me and not be so greedy with them, since me and my sex life were not on speaking terms. We both laughed and drank the rest of the bottle as we wound down the reality of another day.

When I got home, I plopped down on the couch, grateful for Betty's levity and for holding up the mirror in which to see myself. Why was I OK with a nonexistent sex life? I couldn't feel anything related to my own sexuality anymore. I had no interest, little curiosity, and most of the time felt pretty unbothered about its absence. It was rare that I even felt called to masturbate, let alone initiate sex with my partner. Who was I? What was I missing? Was my relationship OK?

In the days and weeks that followed, I started talking with more friends about it. My friend group is not shy and we talk about sex with ease, but it hadn't been a regular conversation for a long time. A few were unhappily married, and one was gearing up for divorce. Another was on a fertility journey to become a single mom by choice. A few of my other friends had stopped dating to focus on work or because they were tired of the apps and taking a break. Most of us, in an unconscious pact of solidarity, were in a sexless funk!

One friend, in a somber tone, asked, "What does it feel like to be disconnected from your sexuality? Something in that resonates, but I wouldn't know if I was disconnected from it." My immediate response was, "It feels like deadness. Like a part of the lifeblood that makes me who I am no longer flows. Like an abandoned piece of earth, cluttered with the dead and dried-out leaves of a once colorful, thick, flowering garden that was once nourished, and now can't even hold a drop of moisture. It has been unattended for so long; just an abandoned void, living inside of me."

It sounds dire and intense, but that's how it felt. My friends nodded; my story seemed to resonate with what they'd been feeling. After hearing myself say this out loud, I decided I'd had enough. I was going to reconnect with my sexuality. The sexual disconnect left me at odds with so many other parts of myself. I didn't feel whole, embodied, or alive. I felt numb and flat—not dissociative, just not very dynamic. My creativity was tapped out, I wasn't cooking anymore (a hobby I once loved) or enjoying the little moments. It wasn't just that I was disconnected from my sexuality, I was disconnected from myself.

This book was born out of my search for a way through that deadness, the emptiness, the disconnection. This is likely where your story begins, too. Picking up this book means you've felt it, just like me. Or something like it. I hope your path takes you back to yourself, and into a relationship with sex that feels fulfilling once again.

Before you begin, a few caveats about this book.

Its organization is designed into three parts to explore (1) what could be happening within yourself contributing to your shift in desire, (2) what could be happening within the context of a relationship, and (3) to help you construct some tangible steps and starting points. However, your relationship with desire might not be impacted by just one thing, so you may recognize parts of yourself across various chapters. This is to be expected because desire is a complicated tapestry. Feel free to take what feels meaningful to you and leave the rest.

Each chapter is its own possibility for self-exploration, reflecting a question you might have asked yourself as you pondered the reason or reasons for your lost desire. They cover some of the most common themes therapists see in practice, such as shame, healing from trauma, relational inequities, sexual entitlement, and desire discrepancy, but they are not meant to be an exhaustive list, as there are a multitude of reasons for a disconnect with desire. Each chapter ends with a section titled Pleasure Points to help you synthesize its main takeaways. Feel free to skip to the end if you're not quite sure if a chapter is relevant to you. Following the Pleasure Points are self-reflection questions designed to help you explore each topic further as it relates to you (or not).

This book is meant to help you think dimensionally about your relationship with sex, your beliefs about it, and how you negotiate boundaries. Returning to a life filled with desire often requires more than one adjustment, sometimes within yourself and other times within a relationship. As eager as you may be to find solutions, please give yourself patience and grace as you explore your truth and your options. As with sex itself, trying to rush an outcome is likely to leave you disappointed.

Over the course of my nearly twenty years of experience in this field, I have had the great privilege of speaking with thousands of people about their relationships with sex. To protect their confidentiality and to highlight how common various themes are in this work, each case example in this book is a composite of several people's stories. No single example reflects any one client's or person's story exactly.

I am not a physician, so I do not discuss any of the very real reasons for a change in desire that are outside my scope of practice as a psychologist and sex therapist: medical issues, pregnancy and birth, side effects of medication, fluctuating hormones, the arc of peri- to postmenopause (aside from my personal experience), pain during sex that has a physical cause, diet, exercise, and so on. Even if you resonate with what is in this book, I highly encourage you to work with a physician or naturopathic doctor or other qualified medical professional to rule out or treat any underlying medical concern that may be contributing to changes in your libido or felt sense of pleasure.

Also, this book does not cover the spectrum of asexuality. While some folks who feel disconnected from desire do wonder if they are asexual, and may be so, I do not go into depth about it because my aim is to help you *reconnect* with your sexuality and assumes you are looking to reestablish a connection with desire that was once there. For more reading on asexuality, the book *ACE: What Asexuality*

Reveals about Desire, Society, and the Meaning of Sex by Angela Chen is excellent.

This book may rouse some difficult feelings. While that may be uncomfortable, to feel pleasure, we have to sort through emotions, and sometimes that brings discomfort or pain. If you're feeling activated or like parts of this book are too much, please take a break and take care of yourself. This book isn't going anywhere and will be here when you're ready to pick it up again.

Part 1

What's Going On with Me?

Loss of desire is often driven by individual variables, even though some of those variables are the result of interactions within a relationship. This section addresses some of the most common individual psychological themes that can impede desire and arousal, starting with shame and moving through topics such as identity, trauma, burnout, numbness, or avoidance, and feeling angry or resentful. Nothing here is meant to assign blame. Rather, these topics are meant to invite intentional introspection into circumstances that may predate your current dip in desire or are part of a dynamic cause and ripple effect.

Looking inward can empower you to find some control as you move forward. As I reflected on my own sexual journey, it was clear there were some things I brought to the dynamic that had nothing to do with my partner and some that were born in the relationship with my partner. Nonetheless, they were my responsibility to address, at least initially. We can't control our partners. What we can do is look at our part.

Chapter 1

Am I Broken?

Two of the most frequent questions people bring to sex therapy are "Am I normal?" and "Am I broken?" These two questions are really two sides of the same coin: a feeling of shame—a fear of being unlovable or undesirable. At its core, shame, or the fear of being bad or broken, is about relational safety: whether you have (or will have) a sense of security in your primary relationship(s). These worries can lead people to wonder, "Am I safe in this relationship?" "If I am truly myself, will my partner really love me?" "Am I even lovable?" "If I really want a threesome, am I bad?" This fear is often a quiet whisper of the true, deep fear that we will end up alone.

For many folks, their sexual relationships are rife with shame, and this is often a threat to pleasure and relational safety because it inhibits intimacy and convinces you that you are inherently unworthy and unlovable. Shame can corrupt your sense of self and convince you that you are bad. Not that you did a bad thing (which is guilt), but that you at your *core* are bad, wrong, broken. Oof. Shame is rough.

Back to the question "Am I broken?" The short answer is of course not! The long answer will continue throughout this chapter and the whole book. Your relationship with sex, desire, pleasure—whatever brought you here—has no standing on your value and worthiness as a person. Finding out what happened to your sex life starts with honesty and some truths that may increase your frustration before helping you arrive at a solution. That is to be expected, as the only way *to* is *through*. As you read, you might even consider any discomfort you feel as necessary, to move you away from the helplessness or ambivalence you may have felt impeded by to discover a life of passion and vitality.

CASE STUDY

Billie came to my office on a bright summer's day, though her demeanor was anything but bright. Her shoulders curled forward, and her voice was quiet, as if to hide from her shame. She described growing up in a high-control religious environment, in a community where her family was prominent and well-known. Billie's cousin, a man seven years her senior, began sexually abusing her when she was five, and her family's response was to blame her for being "suggestive" and to keep her isolated from the rest of the children, to make her "repent" by subjecting her to extra chores. Billie's cousin was sent to an all-male boarding school for the rest of his schooling, and went on to be a high-achieving student who earned much acclaim within their small community. Billie's mother has a short fuse and often criticized her for not getting her chores done "correctly," despite her working extremely hard to "be good." Billie felt like she was always messing up and could not rid herself of the feeling she was bad, dirty, and "broken."

When Billie eventually married her high school sweetheart, she was excited to have her own household, and to have a life that made up for her difficult childhood. Soon after they were married, she and her husband left the high-control religion and moved to Los Angeles. Sex with him was "nice," and he didn't judge her for her cousin's abuse. Billie knew her husband was safe for her and she wanted to "give him" a good sex life. She enjoyed sex with him, but what she liked about it was that she seemed to be making him happy. She hadn't thought of sex as something for herself to enjoy, and she'd had an orgasm only a few times.

As years passed in their marriage, they had two children, and Billie found herself busy in her role as a mother and less interested in sex. She still said yes when her husband initiated it, but felt herself less motivated to be sexual. Her husband felt her lack of interest and told her he wanted her to want it and to initiate sex more. She obliged for a while. But she "felt weird" being the person to initiate sex because was that something she "should do?" She didn't have a lot of spare time, and by the time the kids were tucked up in bed, she was exhausted. One day, Billie's husband broke down crying as he thought she didn't desire him anymore. He wondered if she was having an affair. Billie was shocked! She loved her husband so much and only loved him. She wasn't having an affair, but she also wasn't feeling a lot of desire. She looked at me, and with a trembling voice, asked, "Am I broken?"

In the realm of human sexuality, there's a term for how Billie feels: "low desire." Low desire is often misunderstood. Many people understand their desire to be "low" because they are comparing their level of sexual desire to someone else's, or they hear from a partner with higher desire that their level means something is wrong *with them*, resulting in shame. Making these normative comparisons (comparing one's own experience to that of a group of others) is rarely a helpful way to conceptualize one's own relationship with desire. A better metric to consider is whether your desire has changed compared to your baseline. In reality, desire is a dynamic experience and can ebb and flow with time, interest, stress, and so on. Countless individuals and couples have struggled with a decrease in their desire or a discrepancy in desire with their partner, believing that it represents an intrinsic flaw or problem within themselves or their relationships. If you're feeling broken or not normal because of the desire you aren't feeling, it is important to challenge the language of "low" desire, especially if it's being weaponized against you. Instead, reframing it as "lower"—perhaps than you'd like—can help you explore the multifaceted nature of human sexual desire with a more open mind.

Desire is a complex interplay of physical, psychological, and social factors. When woven together, these factors dictate the motivation to have sex. Those factors are biological (including hormones, neurotransmitters, and overall health), psychological (like mental health, emotions, self-esteem, and past experiences), as well as social and cultural (like relationships, religious beliefs, and cultural norms). When we use terms like "low desire," it implies that there is a static and normative continuum of desire from low to average to high. But sexual desire is fluid and dynamic, and when it is pathologized as low (read: insufficient) it can create an unnecessary and unhelpful wedge between a person and their sexuality. It is *natural* for desire to fluctuate over time. Having lower desire is not necessarily indicative of a problem with you or your relationship, but rather is pointing to an expected aspect of human sexuality.

A common cause shaping our worries about "low desire" is a desire discrepancy between partners in a relationship. Partners often experience different levels of sexual desire and at different times. Believing that you and your partner should desire sex at the same intensity and rate can lead to frustration, fears of inadequacy, and conflict. You're not hungry, thirsty, or tired at the same rate or time—so why would sexual desire be any different?

Causes of Lower Desire

Let's take a closer look at the psychological, social, and cultural aspects of desire. Some psychological aspects include your relationship with your body image, previous trauma, anxiety, depression, or stress, all of which can impact or amplify desire. Social and cultural factors may be perceived social expectations, norms from your culture or religion, and scripts from pop culture or movies, which are also key influencers. Added pressures about body image and appearance can leave you feeling shame about yourself, at odds with desire, and extra vulnerable or uncomfortable when naked or in your own skin.

Relationship dynamics can play an important role. Unresolved conflicts, impasses in communication, emotional distance, or questions about trust can temporarily reduce a partner's desire. If you're fighting with your partner about things big or small and there is insufficient repair, that can lead to slumps. It may not seem obvious at first, but a lack of adequate repair can often lead to loss of respect, loss of trust, and a loss of emotional safety. That's not to say that all desire is due to a shift in the relationship or that the relationship is doomed if desire fades. With resolution of the relationship dynamics, desire often finds its way back.

There are many medical and biological factors that can disrupt desire as well. Changes in hormones, medical conditions, and some medications (such as antidepressants) can impact desire directly, or can have other symptoms or side effects, such as fatigue, lack of sleep, or pain.

Major life events can temporarily reduce desire such as becoming a parent, changing or losing a job, or taking care of elderly parents. Losing a loved one is accompanied by the stress of managing the loss, or there can be unresolved conflict or relational strife with the deceased person resulting in trauma symptoms appearing upon their death, as well as grief. All of these aspects of life are part of being human.

Gender, Shame, and Control

Through the last several centuries, society has perpetuated the erroneous and damning misconception that people assigned female at birth (AFAB) have inherently less desire than people assigned male at birth (AMAB). This harmful notion stems from an oversimplified and problematic comparison between two sexes on a gender binary. As such, women's desire is often unfairly compared to male desire, with an assumption that male desire is the norm. This is problematic for several reasons. It overlooks the inherent diversity in individual desire; simplifies and reduces complex emotional and physical factors related to each person's temperament, experiences, and expected oscillations in desire; and ignores the vital role of context and culture, especially as it relates to gender role socialization. It also makes invisible anyone who falls outside of the gender binary and continues a pattern of erasure toward already marginalized groups of people.

Research on human sexual response reveals that people AFAB and AMAB share similar physiological processes and behaviors related to desire, arousal, and orgasm. In her book *Come as You Are*, Emily Nagoski famously and repeatedly wrote that genitals are "all the same parts, just organized in different ways."[1] Patterns of desire vary wildly among people of all genders; gender does not define our preferences. However, societal expectations have long enforced gender roles that place men in the position of pursuing sex, and women as the passive recipients of men's desire. This deeply ingrained social script has helped lead to a default and completely erroneous perception of women as having lower desire than men. Recognizing that peoples' desires can vary widely, regardless of sex, gender, or sexual orientation, is the first step toward a more inclusive and accurate understanding of your own sexuality and that of any partner.

Another dangerous myth is the notion that women are inherently responsible for responding to men's sexual desires and that any deviation from this norm is seen as "broken" or unacceptable. Historically, the patriarchy—a system of power that rules men as supreme—has played a significant role in shaping societal perceptions of female sexuality, and it has created a narrative that women exist to please men sexually but do not have their own desire. This juxtaposition is intentional, as it disempowers women and undermines their sexual autonomy.

Of course, women's sexuality does not exist for the benefit of men, much to the dismay of patriarchal ideology. The origins of patriarchy involved controlling female sexuality, to procure power and the transfer of wealth among men.[2] It's no surprise that as patriarchy evolved, so did the belief that women's sexuality existed for male pleasure. Power corrupts, and in this case, commodified women's bodies and co-opted their pleasure. For so many men—good men, men you love and who love you—the conditioning of patriarchy has been so unconsciously absorbed that they do not understand the ways it has manifested in their worldview, relationships, and sex lives. This notion does not speak for the desire of women and people AFAB who do not have sex with men. A woman's sexuality is hers alone, and is not a measure of her worth or social currency. With whom (if anyone) and how she chooses to share her sexuality is up to her alone. However, expectations and feelings of obligation connected to sexual entitlement have been shown to have the opposite relationship with sexual desire.[3] No wonder! If sex feels like a chore or an obligation, it is likely to be deprived of pleasure. If the sex someone is having is not good sex, they are less ready to want more. Why would someone desire something that does not bring them pleasure?

A cornerstone of healthy and fulfilling sex is autonomy and consent. All partners should be free to express their desires and boundaries without having to capitulate to predefined gender roles. Women and people AFAB, like people of all genders, have a wide range of valid sexual desires and orientations, regardless of whether they align with traditional, heteronormative, or patriarchal expectations. Healthy sexual relationships are built on a foundation of mutuality, honesty, transparent communication, and respect for each other's limits.

A critical tool of patriarchy is shame, and it has been confounded with female sexuality for thousands of years. Shaming women for their sexual desires, or lack of desire to reciprocate a man's desire, has long been a strategy for engineering control over women and their sexuality. Publicly shaming women serves to keep their access to resources limited, keeping them in a state of insecurity and dependent on men's approval. While equality movements have shifted women's rights, many tenets of sexism are still alive and well, especially related to sexual interests and autonomy. In a patriarchy, financial and social resources are gatekept by men. There is an often unconscious and sometimes conscious hope that a woman who feels inherently flawed (whether she wants more or less sex than her partner believes she should want) will keep a dynamic in place where her partner is the authority over her sexuality and she is the identified problem. Countless women self-refer to sex therapy because their (often male) partner has threatened to leave them because their desire is lower than his. Patriarchal coding around power, authority, and sexuality is often a culprit when it comes to desire undiscovered or disconnected.

Stop pathologizing yourself. *You are not broken.*

If you have any doubts, please read that last sentence again.

Fluctuations in desire are to be expected; there is no one-size-fits-all approach. What can feel like lower desire to one person may be another person's higher desire experience. And conversely, what might feel like higher desire to someone may feel like a dip to someone else. Stop comparing yourself to others or to an expected group norm. Instead of viewing yourself as broken, pause and re-approach the way you view yourself. Speak to yourself with compassion and without judgment. Perhaps you've found your way to this book because your partner has expressed concern in the discrepancy of your desire, or because *you* want a different sex life. If either is true, a compassionate self-view can help you find answers throughout this book, accompanied by some action steps that feel empowering, authentic, and sustainable.

Instead of labeling yourself or your partner as "low desire," meet each other with open and empathetic communication. Discussing your needs for emotional, physical, and sexual intimacy can help bridge the gap and foster greater connection. Shifting away from the idea of brokenness is key to rekindling desire. I invite you instead to focus on enhancing pleasure—of all forms, not just sexual. There will be more on how to do this in chapter 16.

Pleasure Points

- Many people worry if they are "abnormal" or "broken" due to feeling less desire than they want to feel or less desire than they believe they *should* feel, which can lead to fears of being abandoned, undesirable, or unlovable.

- Shame related to sex can wound self-esteem, perpetuate feelings of unworthiness, and make desire feel even less accessible.

- Healthy sex starts with consent, focuses on pleasure, involves communication, and is unique to each individual and their interests. It is not about frequency.

- Difference in desire between partners is common, and should not be internalized as a flaw. It is an inevitable component of human sexuality.

- Harmful myths about gender and desire perpetuate misconceptions, particularly the belief that women inherently have lower desire than men.

Pleasure Reflections

- How do societal expectations and cultural norms influence my perception of my own desire? Am I comparing myself to others? Can I stop?

- What factors in my life (e.g., stress, health, relationship dynamics, unfulfilling sex) might be affecting my current level of desire?

- How do I define healthy sex? And how does this definition align with my personal experiences and values? Where might there be incongruences?

- What role might shame play in my relationship with sex and desire? Do I have shame about my lack of desire? My sexual interests?

Chapter 2

Who Am I?

Many of us take our sense of self for granted. Yet many of my clients, regardless of background, have dimensions of their identity that have not been well explored. This makes sense, as self-exploration is not generally something we're taught when we're young. We just become who we are, and later, when things are bumpy, we might feel compelled to explore how identity plays a role.

This is especially true when it comes to sex, which is often a hotbed of cognitive dissonance and identity conflicts. We don't often think about the relationship between desire and identity, but someone whose identity is in flux or not fully defined may not have a strong sense of what, if anything, turns them on. Sexual desires and activity can be one way someone seeks to understand and define themselves in the absence of a well-formed sense of self. There can also be conflict between how a person sees themselves, or rather, how they *want* to see themselves, and what they like sexually. When a person is not secure in their identity, it is hard to feel integrated, confident, authentic, or safe, which can play an integral role in accessing desire.

So, what is identity? Identity develops from a couple of motivations. First, the human brain doesn't like ambiguity. We develop labels (identities) as a kind of shorthand, so we can better understand ourselves and each other without the difficulty of labored descriptions of who we are, what we like, and why. In other words, the language of identity helps to conserve mental energy and speed up the process of understanding the world around us and our place in it.

The second is to cultivate a sense of belonging. As humans, we seek connection with others. Humans are relational in nature, though to varying degrees. Feeling as if we are members of a group, whether it be our family, coworkers, political party, gender, religious group, and so on, gives us a sense of belonging that contributes to relational safety, connection, and a sense of worthiness and security in the world. Seeking connection is in service of our survival. In groups, such as our families or communities, we have a better chance of being cared and provided for. Resources are obtained by the group, for the group. Members of a group advocate for each other's well-being and that includes making sure the members stay safe and have access to what they need to succeed in life. Procuring and sharing resources is especially important in times of economic difficulty, forming the basis of intragroup (group infighting) and intergroup (fighting a different group or opponent) conflict, evident amongst rivaling sports teams or political parties.

Multiple Identities, One Self

Our self-concept or identity is dynamic. It continually evolves as we change, learn, and grow. We see and define ourselves based on how we see and define others, as well as through the feedback we get from other people about ourselves. This can be a healthy paradigm in which to explore self-expression and authenticity. However, in cultures driven by power hierarchies, safety and worthiness are often over-coupled with identity. In other words, in systems of power (such as patriarchy, racism, or capitalism), those who hold the most are considered to be supreme. This means they have the most protection when it comes to wealth, control, and resources. I'm not saying this is how the world should be, but it is the reality of living in a power and wealth-driven society, and our membership in various in-groups based on our identities can mean the difference between feast or famine. But we don't just have *one* identity or belong to *one* group. Our holistic sense of self is composed of many identities or categorizations that tell us (and others) something about who we are in this world.

Our sense of self is made up of many intersectional identities, including but not limited to our gender identity, gender expression, race, ethnicity, cultural background, religious beliefs, education, socioeconomic status, physical ability, body image, age, mental health, relationship status, and of course, our sexual orientation. Intersectionality,[1] a concept developed and named by Kimberlé Crenshaw, a scholar and civil rights advocate, outlines the multiple factors that shape a person's identity, as well as their experiences (in their bodies, relationships, and the world), privileges, and disadvantages. Each intersecting identity can influence and interact with the others and all influence how we experience pleasure, especially sexual desire and fantasies. For example, a queer woman of color might navigate unique challenges due to the combined effects of sexism, racism, homophobia, and heteronormativity, which could lead to internal conflicts about her own desires or desirability. Similarly, people from a lower socioeconomic background or those with disabilities may face additional stressors and a lack of resources impacting their sexual health and desire. Anyone can be fetishized or sexually objectified, and people in marginalized groups often experience fetishization and sexual exploitation at a higher rate, which may lead to apprehension about sex.

Further, mental health conditions influenced or exacerbated by experiences of discrimination or marginalization can lead to decrease in desire. Erotic minorities (for example, people who enjoy kink, fetishes, nonmonogamy, or other aspects of sex outside the mainstream) may be at greater risk of shame, violence, or risk of being ostracized from groups that do not tolerate sexual expansiveness.

CASE STUDY

Erica was interested in exploring an open relationship with her partner, Nadia. They had discussed feeling curious about nonmonogamy, but Erica feared that being a lesbian was already "too much" as a Christian, and she was grateful her parents and church had accepted her and Nadia. Despite wanting to invite other partners into their sex life, Erica shut down future conversations with Nadia on the topic. Nadia grew frustrated and pleaded with Erica to revisit their options, suggesting they didn't have to tell her family or congregation. Erica was too afraid someone would find out, and ruin her mother's impression of Nadia as a "good girl."

How many identities did you catch? Erica identified as a *woman, lesbian, Christian,* and *monogamous* person. She also identified Nadia (and likely herself) as "good girls," conflating adherence to the rule of monogamy with morality and worthiness. Erica and Nadia grew less and less interested in sex with one another over time, because neither were being authentic in their desires to open the relationship, and both felt they were being asked to hide parts of themselves in order to stay in the good graces of Erica's family.

Take a moment to reflect on your sexual desires and how they relate to the various intersectional parts of your identity by completing the following sentences. Be honest with yourself and use this exercise as an opportunity to deepen your understanding of how different parts of your identity may influence your sexual preferences. If you find that reflecting on your sexual desires brings up more feelings of shame, it's OK to take a break to allow yourself to process what you're uncovering about yourself.

- When I think about my gender identity in relation to my sexual desires, I feel . . .

- My gender expression plays a role in my sexual desires by . . .

- Considering my racial identity, I notice that it affects my sexual desires in the following ways . . .

- When exploring my ethnic background, I find that it influences my sexual desires by . . .

- Reflecting on my cultural background, I recognize that it shapes my sexual desires through . . .

- My religious beliefs impact my sexual desires in the following ways . . .

- Considering my level of education, I see that it has an impact on my sexual desires because . . .

- When thinking about my socioeconomic status, I notice that it influences my sexual desires in the following ways . . .

- My physical abilities affect my sexual desires by . . .
- Reflecting on my body image, I observe that it shapes my sexual desires through . . .
- Considering my age, I find that it influences my sexual desires by . . .
- When reflecting on my mental health, I notice that it impacts my sexual desires because . . .
- My current relationship status plays a role in my sexual desires by . . .
- Exploring my sexual orientation, I recognize that it shapes my sexual desires through . . .

Take your time with each statement, allowing yourself to delve into your thoughts and feelings. This exercise is meant for personal reflection; there are no right or wrong answers. Use it as a tool for greater self-awareness and understanding.

The Cost of Membership

What does intersectionality have to do with dips in desire? Holding a specific identity is like belonging to a club. There are commonalities and usually a shared set of implicit and explicit rules about what sets you apart from other clubs, or in this case, other identities. In order to maintain membership in the club, you agree to comply with the established guidelines. If you decide the group's norms no longer work for you (or never did), issues arise.[2] Either you stay loyal to the group and practice some element of self-abandonment, or stay true to yourself and run the risk of being ostracized from the group. And some identities—such as race, ethnicity, or a disability—cannot be abandoned, so what happens then? Our identities shape our experience of belonging or exclusion, and if our sense of belonging is threatened, our minds can engage in some interesting mental gymnastics to find a way to balance what is authentic with what allows us to feel safe or included. This bind between authenticity and belonging can lead to compartmentalized identities, or identities that become isolated from our consciousness or expression. People may develop self-loathing around an identity or deny that it exists. They may develop hatred toward others who maintain a specific identity, or exempt themselves from believing that certain aspects of an identity apply to them, too. We may cut off or distance ourselves from these parts of our identities in an effort to minimize conflict or avoid the effects of stigma from others, or align ourselves with the parts of our identities that judge those elements that we do not wish to be true.

Conflicts often arise between your erotic identity and other identities that are part of you, such as ethnicity or religion. Those conflicts then form an intricate web of denial, inhibition, disavowal, low self-acceptance, and shame when it comes to desire, fantasy, and sexual behavior. So many identity-based memberships come with prohibitions around sex, forcing you into ties of loyalty between yourself and your community. Staying loyal to the group often means practicing some element of self-abandonment, which creates an existential crisis. It can take a long time to realize that your sense of belonging with people you care about may be contingent on something as arbitrary as whether you like stinging sensations on your bum or a little role play with your orgasms.

When two parts of your identity are in conflict, it is common to shut off parts of yourself in exchange for the safety, protection, and connection of your community. This practice is called compartmentalization, and it can help you feel safe within a group at the expense of stunting your desire. On the flip side, an identity that is without shame and is integrated (meaning all parts are accepted) can foster community with other people (other groups), more self-exploration and intimacy with others, open and transparent communication, and a sense of wholeness. Not to mention the untapped pleasure potential!

Humans crave authenticity in their identity. When we deny a part of ourselves, such as keeping a sexual desire or interest at bay, we inhibit opportunities for growth, pleasure, and true connection. Disavowing parts of oneself can render a chronic feeling of being stuck in a pattern of self-abandonment and resentment. You might wonder just how safe it is to stay in a group if the price of membership is your authenticity. And there are some groups, as discussed earlier, that we cannot just opt out of. However, trusting the process of self-acceptance and integration requires a leap of faith and often comes with real consequences if you choose to step away from the group's protection and stake a claim in your own authenticity. Especially when it comes to our very charged, very morally constructed paradigm around sex, even in the twenty-first century. If it does not feel realistic to depart from one group altogether, building relationships within a new community can help foster integration, belonging, safety, and connection.

People Like *Me* Don't Do *That*

What does an erotic identity conflict look or sound like? It is often a belief that people like you shouldn't enjoy or be curious about the sexual fantasies or behaviors that spark something in you.

CASE STUDY

Christine loved her husband Paul, but hated that he watched porn, and really hated that he asked her to watch it with him. They talked about spicing up their marriage, but this was the only idea he contributed to their small list of options. Paul insisted that porn was an appetizer for him, and pleasure with Christine was his main focus, but Christine couldn't shake the idea that they needed an "appetizer" to get in the mood. She thought erotic material was for people who didn't love each other or who had "bad morals," but admittedly she was curious about what Paul watched. Was he into BDSM? Group sex? Something else? Christine did have some fantasies about rough sex, but as a feminist, she refused to let herself go down that path—in porn or reality. There was enough violence toward women in porn and in the world. She wouldn't participate in something so misogynistic, as that would make her a "bad" feminist.

Seeing a theme yet? Good or bad. Right or wrong. Moral or amoral. In or out of the group. Christine's identities as a woman and a feminist prevented her from exploring even erotic material related to her ethics, or new scripts with her husband that may have opened the door to deeper intimacy. She, like many people, was afraid that her fantasy and play life would somehow contaminate her worthiness as a feminist, a woman, and likely as a human.

This is not an exhaustive list, but here are additional examples of erotic identity conflicts.

1. Someone identifying as asexual feels pressure to conform (from a partner or society) to the expectation of sexual desire, leading to internal conflict.

2. Someone wanting to explore kinks or fetishes feels held back by internalized shame.

3. One partner wanting to explore nonmonogamy, while the other is not interested in anything but monogamy.

4. Someone identifying as LGBTQIA+ struggles to reconcile their sexual orientation with cultural or religious expectations that prioritize heteronormativity.

5. Someone wanting sex more frequently, or with more partners, than they believe is acceptable, as dictated by religious or cultural expectations.

6. Someone with a foot fetish thinking that liking feet makes them "gross," because feet are "gross."

Morality, Worthiness, and Sex

Do any of the groups you belong to (i.e., gender, religion, age, etc.) require you to deprioritize pleasure or deny it altogether in order to be seen as a good person? Do any of your identities apply conditions or assign morality depriving your pleasure? This can lead to a decrease in desire or aversion to sex itself. No one needs to *earn* pleasure. To feel pleasure is part of being human. That is, not sex with another person, which requires consent—but *pleasure* is something all humans get to experience and of which we are worthy.

Now let's explore your relationship with pleasure, both nonsexual and sexual. How do you prioritize pleasure in your life?

Many people have been conditioned to believe that they have to earn pleasure, or that if they experience or prioritize pleasure, *they are not good people*. This is a conflation of morality, worthiness, and sexuality. But these topics are not so black and white. The experience of power, self-worth, identity, and belonging dictate many folks' perception of who *should* be able to have different kinds of pleasure, as well as how or when they *should* experience it. If they depart from that predetermined path, then they are *bad*. If they adhere to the path, they are *good*.

Enter disgust. Disgust plays an important role in sex, as it serves as a gatekeeper for our physical self, our perception of ourselves, or our self-concept.[3] If you believe a certain kind of sex is incongruent with the kind of sex you, according to your identities, *should* like, you may feel disgust toward that sexual thought or activity.

CASE STUDY

Joy was enamored with her partner, but came into a session distressed because he wanted to try anal sex. She shrieked, "No one *I know* does that! I'm not a porn star! Why would he think I would do that? Gross."

It's clear that Joy is disgusted about what people might do or see in porn, as she immediately created an us/them dichotomy where people who are sex workers have anal sex and people who are not sex workers do not. This is a common form of internalized misogyny and many women are conditioned to uphold patriarchal ideas about sexual purity to maintain their social standing. Like many women, Joy unconsciously positioned herself in a higher status by devaluing a sexual activity as disgusting, and thereby implying the same of sex workers.

Disgust, shame, judgment, and avoidance are all close bedfellows when it comes to balancing the demands of our identities with our safety, worthiness, and belonging in the world. Sexual double standards are another societal tool to maintain social hierarchy and a prevailing culprit in the assessment of lower desire in women.[4] Slut-shaming has been a profoundly effective and abhorrent tool of patriarchy and purity culture, robbing many people, especially women, of the chance to explore their fullest sexual desires. This conditioning starts early in life, and can be an important variable to explore if you are trying to understand why your desire has changed.

I invite you to consider how you may be holding onto moral judgments about yourself, or other people, based on a desired frequency for sex, number of partners you/they have or want, the nature of your/their fantasies, and the way you/they express gender and sexual identities. Might there be anything holding you back? What would happen if you stopped "should-ing" yourself?

Pleasure Points

- There is often a strong relationship between desire, identity, and the impact of belonging to various groups or communities.

- A person's evolving identity can affect their sexual desires and behaviors.

- Intersectional identities that shape an individual's sense of self can influence how much permission they give themselves to be sexual.

- Adherence to group norms can lead to compartmentalized identities and hinder personal growth and pleasure.

Pleasure Reflections

- How have your various intersecting identities, such as gender, sexual orientation, and cultural background, shaped your own understanding of sexuality and desire?

- Reflect on a situation where you felt torn between staying true to yourself and conforming to group expectations regarding sexuality. How did this loyalty bind impact your authenticity?

- Can you recall a personal experience where societal norms or group expectations influenced your attitudes toward sexuality? How did this affect your ability to express your true desires and find pleasure?

- Think about situations in your life where external expectations or your own beliefs may have conflicted with your exploration of sexual desires. How did these factors influence your ability to authentically engage with and express your sexuality?

Chapter 3

Why Can't I Get Over It?

Healing after any kind of trauma, and especially sexual trauma, requires perpetual effort. In contrast to the narratives projected in mainstream media about what is expected of survivors, healing is not linear. Healing is often messy and imperfect, and there is no one right way to do it. There are many variables that shepherd someone onto the path of recovery, such as the amount of support they have from personal and professional communities, access to resources like a therapist or legal assistance, their history of trauma preceding the event, preexisting mental health conditions, the sensitivity and competence of any professional involved, cultural beliefs about sexual violence, and so on, which vary from survivor to survivor. Each survivor's healing journey is unique—and so is their relationship with sex.

The Many Layers of Sexual Trauma

Sexual entitlement and the pervasive presence of sexual violence in relationships have a significant potential impact on desire. Sexual trauma, coupled with a culture of sexual entitlement and a media landscape rife with sexual violence, can shape and alter your experience of desire. Each person responds differently to such experiences. For some survivors, the impact of sexual trauma is a decrease in desire, while for others, desire may paradoxically increase. Your interest in sex may fluctuate in response to traumatic experiences, swinging between periods of low or no desire and higher desire. These responses can feel confusing but they are common and natural. The unconscious mind is aiming to control a situation (sex) in which you were once physically or emotionally overpowered.

CASE STUDY

Avery had worked hard to have a positive relationship with sex after she was sexually assaulted in college. After the assault, she was incessantly slut-shamed and harassed, which became a predictable and infuriating part of her day with no one on campus taking her outcry seriously. She transferred to a new college and waited five years before considering sex again. Avery felt robbed of the opportunity to explore her sexuality.

By her mid-thirties, Avery had embraced her sexuality and was thrilled to meet Ben, whose libido matched hers. Ben felt like a safe partner for Avery, who had a hard time letting people in. She wasn't one to tell people, especially men she dated, that she had been raped. After the victim blaming she'd endured, she no longer wanted people to know what had happened to her or to run the risk of not feeling supported again. A little over a year into their relationship, one of Avery's good friends was raped by a new dating partner. Avery leaped to her side and supported her in a way she wished the friends she'd had at college would have done for her.

Ben started to feel slighted because Avery was spending so much time with her friend. In a heated conversation, Ben told Avery that she should stop spending so much time with her friend, because her friend was "clearly trying to get attention" and her claim was probably a "false allegation," since her date "seemed like a nice guy" when they'd double dated a few weeks before the assault. Avery immediately felt nauseous. She didn't expect Ben to have a such a skeptical view of sexual violence, and while he immediately apologized for being "snarky," Avery noticed a big shift in her desire for Ben, which also become noticeable to Ben over the following months. Avery didn't know what happened, because she talked with Ben about his comment and her past experience. He apologized again, and reiterated he was just upset they hadn't been spending as much time together, and didn't mean to minimize her friend's pain. Their sex life had been so full, but now Avery felt less interested in sex. She asked, "Why can't I get over this?"

Understanding Sexual Trauma and Desire

Sexual trauma encompasses a broad spectrum of experiences, ranging from overt,[1] such as sexual assault, to covert, as in coercion or noncontact sexual violations, such as sexual harassment at work, catcalling, inappropriate sexual jokes, cyber harassment, or being exposed to pornography or sexually explicit conversations as a child. Survivors of sexual trauma may carry the weight of their experiences into their intimate lives, and this can profoundly affect their relationship with desire.

Covert sexual trauma, characterized by subtle violations of boundaries and trust, can erode a person's sense of safety and autonomy just as much as overt trauma. This can manifest in a diminished desire for intimate connection, as survivors may have anxiety, struggle to feel safe, or have a heightened fear of vulnerability. Both overt and covert sexual trauma can have a direct impact on desire, ranging from an aversion to sex to the reclamation of sexual agency as a form of empowerment. Both are forms of protection for a survivor whose autonomy has been overruled. Aversion keeps the survivor from being in a situation that may result in feelings of helplessness or powerlessness, whereas engaging in sexual behavior can be one way to evoke a sense of personal power to counter feelings of vulnerability.

Sexual trauma doesn't only affect desire, but its impact reverberates through many dimensions of a person's life, profoundly influencing brain development, identity formation, social relationships, romantic partnerships, spirituality, and one's relationship with their body and sovereignty. Trauma impacts a survivor's overall well-being. Let's take a closer look at each one of these effects.

IMPACT ON THE BRAIN

The effects of sexual trauma on brain development can be profound and extensive, particularly in regions associated with emotion regulation, memory processing, and stress response. Trauma can cause alterations in neural pathways that lead to heightened nervous system arousal, hypervigilance, or even dissociation as adaptive coping mechanisms, in nonsexual and sexual moments. These changes can contribute to the development of conditions like post-traumatic stress disorder (PTSD), impacting not only the survivor's mental health but also how they engage in healthy, intimate relationships.

IDENTITY

Sexual trauma can disrupt the process of identity formation as survivors grapple with a profound sense of violation and betrayal. The trauma may introduce a distorted self-perception, characterized by shame, guilt, and a fragmented or compartmentalized sense of self. Some of the ways you might recognize this can be having a pervasive sense of not knowing who you really are, feeling like different people in different contexts, feeling unsure of a coherent narrative or direction in your life, feeling chronically empty, having a difficult time sustaining meaningful relationships, not knowing what you really want, need, or how you feel, or feeling plagued with self-doubt. Survivors may be inclined to blame themselves, or see themselves as inherently unworthy of love, respect, protection, or safety.

SOCIAL RELATIONSHIPS

Survivors can have trouble forming and maintaining social connections. The fear of judgment, isolation, or triggering experiences can lead to social withdrawal. Building trust in relationships becomes a complex task, as survivors may struggle with vulnerability and the potential of being retraumatized. It may require intentional effort to navigate friendships and family dynamics and create a supportive network. Sometimes creating distance or cutting off contact is the only way for a survivor to protect themselves.

ROMANTIC RELATIONSHIPS

As Judith Herman writes, "Recovery can take place only within the context of relationships; it cannot occur in isolation."[2] While this is true—romantic relationships can feel like a healing respite for a survivor—the impact of sexual trauma on romantic relationships can be profound and can affect both the survivor and often their partner. Intimacy can become a source of anxiety, triggering memories of the trauma or causing the survivor to disconnect from physical and emotional closeness. Partners may need to engage in open communication, empathy, and a shared commitment to healing to foster a relationship that supports both individuals' needs. Survivors in a partnership may find it difficult to assert boundaries or fear they are unworthy of love, protection, or care. Conversely, a partner may inadvertently or intentionally engage in secondary re-victimization through insensitive, hurtful, or undereducated remarks. Some survivors may require a sense of control and have a difficult time allowing themselves to feel vulnerable with their partner or fully trusting themselves or their partner in the relationship.

SEXUAL DESIRE

Sexual trauma can significantly alter one's experience of sexual desire.[3] While some survivors may encounter a decrease in desire due to associations between intimacy and trauma, as mentioned earlier, others may experience a paradoxical increase as a way of regaining a sense of control. Navigating these complexities requires a nuanced approach that prioritizes consent, communication, and the gradual rebuilding of trust, not only with others but with your own body and desires.

For survivors, the body can become a battleground. What can feel pleasurable in one moment may feel inaccessible or even distressing in others, and this can result in dissociation as a form of protection. Reclaiming pleasure, especially sexual pleasure, in your body often involves patience and compassion as you explore bodily sensations.

Social and cultural factors can also exacerbate the complexity of post-traumatic desire. Pressure from partners to get over it, dismiss your experience, or to prioritize their pleasure—because *they* weren't the person who hurt you—can feel reminiscent of the sexual entitlement that fueled the sexual violence perpetrated against you. Seeing reminders of sexual violence in media, hearing about it from friends or loved ones, or experiencing reminders of your own trauma, no matter where you are in your healing, can elicit a shift in your relationship with desire. How long the shift lasts depends on the intensity of the trigger, the support at your disposal, and your coping strategies.

SPIRITUALITY

In the aftermath of sexual violence, it is common for survivors to feel an impact in their spiritual lives. The violation of personal boundaries and breach of autonomy can lead to a loss in trust in the world and an existential questioning that can drive a reevaluation of their relationship with a higher power. This is especially true when the perpetration occurred within the context of spiritual or religious relationships, or by another person in the survivor's spiritual or religious community who exploited their trust. In some cases, an unearned level of trust is reserved for people in religious communities, trusting that shared beliefs are proof another person is without the capacity for or interest in exploitation. When that proves to be untrue, it can shake their beliefs about the safety of not only the abusive person but also their religious or spiritual community, and sometimes even their faith. Conversely, other survivors lean into the solace they find within spiritual practices and religious places, feeling protected by their faith's safety. Some survivors may find themselves to be wavering between states of belief: investigation, questioning, and feeling affirmed. This can complicate desire, as sexuality can have spiritual roots and meaning for some folks who believe in sex as a spiritual connection, which can lead to desire-related ambivalence or distress.

BODILY SOVEREIGNTY

Perhaps one of the crueler impacts of sexual violence is disconnection from your own body and bodily sovereignty. Bodily sovereignty means that each person has the right to express agency, autonomy, and self-governance (free will) within and with their bodies. Sexual violence communicates the opposite to the victim—it demands that the victim's sovereignty be subjugated to the will of the perpetrator, and the result for survivors is often feeling as if their body (and their wants, needs, limits, and experiences in it) come second to the wants and needs of others. As a result, survivors may have difficulty setting boundaries, knowing or expressing desires, prioritizing their own agency, practicing self-care, and asserting self-advocacy. It can even limit how well a survivor knows what they want or need.

New Pokes, Same Old Wound

So, why is it hard to heal? Because survivors are often not given the grace, support, justice, or empathy they need to heal and feel restored. Healing from sexual violence is an uphill, zigzagging effort, which most survivors endure on their own.

Not to mention, on a systemic level, our society supports sexual violence. At every turn, survivors are questioned, their efforts at justice thwarted, and their characters misrepresented and blamed, and then when it comes to future sexual activity, they are expected to demonstrate the *right* amount of desire in the *right* contexts, without question and without loading a new partner with the burden of proving they are safe enough. On top of that, our society tolerates rape culture, slut-shaming, and victim blaming, which largely go unchallenged or are even overtly supported, resulting in survivors being bombarded with examples of sexual entitlement, such as a date expecting sex because they paid for your dinner. Sounds hot and steamy, right? Not so much.

In the astutely titled book *The Sexual Alarm System: Women's Unwanted Response to Sexual Intimacy and How to Overcome It*, Judith Leavitt outlines how many women periodically withdraw from sexual desire and intimacy, as a result of constant alerts felt in their bodies regarding sexual entitlement and violence.[4] She outlines the following six specific triggers with one's partner that can elicit a sexual shutdown.

- Aggressive touch that signals sex is imminent
- Touch that is perceived to mean that her partner wants sex
- Any kind of touch or movement that is unexpected or startling
- Vicariously witnessing a violation (e.g., hearing about a sexual assault on the news)
- A look from her partner she interprets as sexual or objectifying
- Sounds that imply desire or objectification

The same stimuli may not always be triggering to the same person or in the same context. And some women may experience desire in response to these stimuli. What constitutes sexual alarm in a given scenario is subjective to that person and that moment. There can be other triggers, too; this is not an exhaustive list. Survivors may experience heightened sensitivity to these stimuli, given that their body has already processed the threat or reality of sexual boundary violations.

CASE STUDY

Inga loved sex, so she was surprised one day when her partner initiated sex, she snapped at him. Her partner was loving and kind, and had never crossed her sexual boundaries, yet she felt alienated from any inkling of desire in response to his bid. She was sexually abused as a child, but did not typically feel heightened emotions or triggers that reminded her of it, as she had been in therapy extensively. This felt different, not like her usual reminders.

Later, when Inga sat down to journal, she recounted her day and tried to identify what set her off. She recalled walking to work and getting a coffee. The man behind her in line made a comment about her outfit, and she remembered feeling creeped out because his gaze lingered. Nothing at work seemed out of the ordinary, but she remembered overhearing two male colleagues talking about their weekend, and heard one say they'd had a one-night stand, but the woman he hooked up with didn't know it was going to be for one night only. On her walk home, she spoke to her good friend who was describing some legislation affecting restrictions on reproductive health care.

Exploring her partner's sexual bid and her strong reaction to it, Inga noted her partner had come up behind her when she was washing dishes. He grabbed her breasts as he hugged her and said, "I'd like to bury my face in these for dessert." He wasn't always so direct in his approach, so this really shocked Inga, and it was on top of those other experiences of hearing language or seeing gestures that felt objectifying and sexually disempowering to her. Not only was she not in the mood, but she was also angry!

Inga was able to recognize, through journaling with intention about her reaction, that her partner's bid felt objectifying and crude to her; it was different than his normal tender and less verbally direct ways of initiating sex. In another relationship, this kind of initiation might be welcomed and not perceived as objectifying. But for Inga, it reminded her not of the abuse she experienced directly, but rather, of how she felt like an object—like her pleasure or experience didn't matter. This happens regularly, when partners have a mismatched bid for sexual play, even if neither are survivors, but it can add an extra layer of aversion for some survivors.

Betrayal

Another common cause of diminished arousal is betrayal. Betrayal trauma can be sexual or nonsexual and take a long time to process, plus there is the added dimension of whether you stay in partnership with the person who betrayed you or move on to a new relationship. Betrayal trauma can linger. The distress of betrayal can look similar to the symptoms of traumatic distress suffered by survivors of sexual violence.

When it comes to infidelity as a form of betrayal, therapist Hope Ray has outlined a new framework for understanding why it can be so painful. She coined the phrase "betrayal violence" to emphasize the effects of behaviors guided by power and control dynamics, which she labels "abusive behavior and communication," to deliberately deceive a partner and violate the fidelity agreements in the relationship.[5] Often, a key component of the trauma of infidelity is knowing your partner went to great lengths to lie in protection of their secret behavior. Therapists who treat betrayal trauma and help couples heal know the deception is often what sends betrayed partners into a fractured state of reality. They don't know who their partner is because they have been lying to them! How can they trust anyone, let alone their partner?

When you stay in a relationship with the person who betrayed you, getting to a new normal may feel like an especially Sisyphean effort. You may want to move through the pain quickly, all the while interacting with a partner who has hurt you, who then minimizes the impact, or insists that their promising words are the only step needed to ensure repair. It can feel maddening and leave you ambivalent about whether you can let your guard down and trust again, or must stay in a position of self-reflection.

Similar to survivors of sexual violence, those who experience betrayal may have divided reactions when it comes to sexual desire, with some betrayed partners experiencing a drop in desire and others an increase. Countless betrayed partners have been told by their (sometimes hopeful, sometimes coercive) partners that being sexual again will help repair the relationship, only to find that desire is nowhere to be found. The betrayed partner may want to have sex, and may yearn for a sense of restored safety that desire may signal, but feel nothing in terms of libido or arousal.

If you are not interested in having sex after a betrayal, listen to the messages from your body as an indication that you do not yet feel safe, secure, or restored in the relationship. Feeling discomfort, apprehension, nausea, muscle tension, and so on, might be an indication that your body may not feel safe enough for sex just yet. More emotional repair may be necessary for you to feel you can surrender into desire. If your partner (or anyone else for that matter) tries to push a timeline for sex that doesn't resonate for you, it can elongate your sexual disconnection, as the lack of attunement to your needs will most likely result in a deeper decline in sexual interest.

For some betrayed partners, there is a desire to connect and an often unconscious attempt to achieve security through the connection of sex. A *sexual bypass*, as it is sometimes called, can give couples an immediate yet superficial feeling of repair, without the real work of repair being done. Couples who try to repair through sex alone may find themselves in an emotional crash down the road, when the problems in the relationship and impact of the betrayal remain unaddressed. Sex is not a cure for unhealthy or incompatible relationship dynamics. Eventually, the deeper emotional work has to be addressed or partners will be faced with the same disappointments and challenges, which can level what may have been a burst of sexual desire and activity into a crater of despair, anxiety, ambivalence, and ultimately decreased desire.

Unless partners make the implicit or explicit agreement to keep their interactions superficial after a betrayal, there is no avoiding the layered and consistent practice of repair if you want to get back to a place where your body truly trusts your partner enough for pleasure to be an option. And, while it is crucial that the betrayed partner participate in repair, if they are leading the charge and overfunctioning (see chapter 11 for more on overfunctioning) for the partner who violated the fidelity agreements, that can increase the discrepancy in sexual desire.

Why Can't I Get Over It?

Sexual trauma or betrayal can render a shock to your system that may forever alter how you exist in your body, relationships, and the world. Returning to an embodied experience (i.e., being present with the sensations in your body) of desire and pleasure can take time, and it is imperative that you set the pace. The body can read the obligation of moving at someone else's pace or expectation as a self-betrayal, prolonging a felt lack of ease when it comes to sex. Healing involves learning to trust others again, but is really about learning to trust yourself. While **none of what happened to you was your**

fault, feeling safe again is an inside job. Trusting others will only get you so far in your healing, because while most are afraid to get hurt, the real fear is that if you get hurt, you won't be able to recover. Building trust in your ability to be OK may take some changes in how you seek out support, resources, and relationships—especially if you stay with someone who violated your trust or boundaries.

Consider your rights and responsibilities to yourself as you lean into sexual empowerment. This list of twenty rights for sexual empowerment is a starting point to think about how you might want to reshape your relationship with sex after sexual trauma or betrayal. Feel free to add your own.

1. **The Right to Your Own Narrative:** You get to define and control your own sexual story, sharing whichever elements of it you wish, as well as when you share them and with whom.

2. **The Right to Consent:** You get to decide whether or not to consent to a sexual activity, freely and without guilt, and to have your boundaries respected.

3. **The Right to Pleasure:** You get to experience sexual pleasure and explore your desires in a way that feels safe enough for you, consensual, and equally prioritized. (The concept of "safe enough" is explored in chapter 7.)

4. **The Right to Communication:** You have the right to be open and honest about your sexual needs, fears, and boundaries with yourself and with partners.

5. **The Right to Self-Exploration:** You have the right to explore your own body, desires, and sexual response without judgment.

6. **The Right to Healthy Relationships:** You have the right to cultivate healthy and supportive sexual relationships that contribute positively to your well-being.

7. **The Right to Boundaries:** You get to establish and communicate clear emotional, physical, and especially sexual boundaries, and have them respected.

8. **The Right to Education:** You have the right to access information and resources about healthy sexuality and relationships to support your healing and your relationship with sex.

9. **The Right to Seek Professional Support:** You have a right to seek therapy or counseling to address any challenges related to your sexuality or relationships, without stigma.

10. **The Right to Celebrate Sexuality:** You get to embrace and celebrate every aspect of your sexuality as a positive aspect of your identity and existence.

11. **The Right to Intimacy:** You have a right to engage in consensual, emotionally and sexually intimate relationships without fear, guilt, or shame.

12. **The Right to Empowerment:** You get to have agency and feel autonomous in your sexual choices, and to take charge of your sexual well-being.

13. **The Right to Mutual Respect:** You have the right to be humanized and treated with respect and dignity by your sexual partners, even in the context of casual sex.

14. **The Right to Safety:** You have the right to define what feels safe enough for you in your safer sex practices, so you can feel secure in your sexual experiences.

15. **The Right to Emotional Support:** You have the right to emotional support from partners and allies as you navigate your sexual healing.

16. **The Right to Say No:** You get to say no to any sexual activity or context at any time without explanation or apology.

17. **The Right to Self-Love:** You have the right to cultivate a practice of self-love and self-acceptance as you reclaim your sexuality, free from the judgment of others.

18. **The Right to Healthy Sexuality Models:** You have the right to access positive and healthy representations of sexuality in media and society.

19. **The Right to Emotional Connection:** You have the right to define, seek out, and cultivate emotional connection in your sexual relationship(s).

20. **The Right to Continued Healing:** You have the right to an ongoing healing process, recognizing that the healing journey both is nonlinear and unique to each person.

Pleasure Points

- Healing from sexual trauma or betrayal is a complex, nonlinear process, and recovery requires some individual work to heal on your own and some healing that can take place only in relationships.

- The impact of sexual trauma, betrayal, or harassment can stretch across several domains of life, including but not limited to the mind and body, identity, social relationships, spirituality, and romantic and sexual relationships.

- Betrayal can produce symptoms and effects similar to those experienced by survivors of sexual violence, due to the deception and dynamics of power and control employed by the betraying partner.

- Your sexuality is yours to nurture and you have many rights to enable an empowered shift in your pleasure.

Pleasure Reflections

- How have societal and media representations shaped your perception of what it means to heal from sexual trauma?

- Reflect on a moment when external factors, such as comments or experiences, triggered a shift in your desire or relationship with sex. How did you navigate it?

- How would you describe your relationship with trust, with others and yourself? How would you like to build more trust with yourself and others? What would be required of you or in the relationship?

- In considering the list of twenty rights for sexual empowerment, which rights resonate with you most as areas where you already feel empowered? Where would you like to feel more empowered?

Chapter 4

Am I Burned-Out?

Connecting to desire is often less about leaning into what turns you on and more about eliminating the things that turn you off.[1] This is especially true when what is disconnecting you from sex is burnout. Often a relevant topic when it comes to people's productivity at work, burnout can have far reaching implications into the rest of your life and act as a thief of your erotic potential and vitality.[2] It's in the name—you are burned-out. What may have been smoldering somewhere in the depths of your being, ready for kindling into a bright hot heat, is now soot, gray and limp without energy.

CASE STUDY

Anne was exhausted all the time, and couldn't remember the last time she had any interest in being sexual, with herself or her partner. In her mid-thirties, Anne worked full-time for an accounting agency and walked dogs on the side for extra money. In 2021, Anne lost her job, and she and her partner went from feeling financially secure to scared about their well-being, living on one salary. Anne's partner's salary covered their expenses, but they had to significantly adjust their lifestyle. Anne canceled her gym membership and started buying groceries in bulk to save money. It took her a year to find another job, and the rapidly changing economy left Anne and her partner playing financial catchup.

One day, Anne's partner looked at her, and said, "Wow, we haven't had sex in three months. Is everything okay?" Anne hadn't even registered the drop in their sexual connection. She was aghast and vowed to herself to change that immediately. Except she didn't think about it again for over a month, when she and her partner were watching a movie with a steamy adult scene. She asked him, "When did we have that conversation about sex—last week?" He smiled, kissed her forehead, and said, "No, a month ago." She was floored and burst out crying. She really wanted to want to have sex, but she just had no desire in her. This was not their normal. Anne asked her partner, "Are we okay?" He affirmed their relationship was not in jeopardy and they made a decision to get to the bottom of why they weren't having sex (and why she wasn't even thinking about it!).

In their first couples' therapy session, it became clear that Anne was working *a lot* and didn't have much time for self-care between work and helping her parents with their healthcare needs. She and her partner had depleted their savings when Anne was laid off, so they were in a rush to restore them and get back on track with their financial goals. Anne's eyes got teary as she realized just how much she had on her plate, and how little time she had for herself over the past few years. There was no quick resolution in sight and Anne felt helpless. She was burned-out and didn't know what to do. Wanting to move back into an erotic space with her partner, Anne decided to take stock in her daily activities and build a schedule that was sustainable and allowed for some intentional rest.

Anne's story is not unique. A chronic culprit of lower desire, burnout can creep up on people. Neither Anne nor her partner recognized their distance from sexual play as a problem, per se, but both were surprised when they realized just how low a priority sex had become. When she realized how much she had taken on, she brought that reality to her partner, and they renegotiated and redistributed the managing of their collective responsibilities. With some new shared agreements, Anne had more time for herself. More time to *feel* like herself. And more time to feel aroused.

I'm Not Burned-Out, Am I?

Burnout can be tricky to spot, since so much praise and social encouragement is attached to achievement. Accolades and financial rewards can float you through the agony of a functional freeze state, when your nervous system is in overdrive while you also feel stuck. The 2021 Work and Well-Being Survey conducted by the American Psychological Association, which polled 1,501 adults, showed that roughly 79 percent of workers reported enduring work-related stress in the month preceding the survey.[3] Of the affected workers, three out of five adults surveyed reported symptoms of burnout, including in three main categories: (1) feeling exhausted, drained, or depleted, (2) feelings of depersonalization or feeling checked out and distant or negative with regard to the demands of work, and (3) feeling a lack of accomplishment or that the efforts put forth are ineffective or meaningless.[4]

Since 2020 and the pandemic, there have been significant changes to the kinds of stressors faced in the workplace. Some professions, including first responders, teachers, therapists, healthcare workers, and essential workers, are more likely to experience burnout than others. For most people, heightened fear around physical well-being, health, money, and political tensions can amplify your financial security or insecurity, leaving you more vulnerable to stressors at work that may otherwise not feel so charged.

Burnout, if left unaddressed, can lead to more significant mental and physical health challenges. Chief among them is a drop in sexual desire.[5] The mind and body are optimized for energy conservation, so feelings and sensations deemed superfluous to our survival often receive fewer resources in times of stress. Even though sex can be a huge stress reliever, it can be hard to allocate the mental or physical energy needed to generate an erotic drive.

If burnout continues for long periods, it can lead to compassion fatigue. Compassion fatigue most often occurs for folks working in helping professions, but it can be experienced in other settings and by stay-at-home parents. It is essentially like burnout amplified, in that it includes emotional and often physical exhaustion, cynicism or apathy, and decreased personal satisfaction in your work. But where it's different and more concerning is that compassion fatigue can also lead to difficulties with concentration that limit a person's effectiveness in their professional and personal roles, cause physical issues like GI concerns, migraines, or sleep disruptions, and hinder a person's capacity for empathy. In a relational context, compassion fatigue can lead to further depleted emotional bandwidth or emotional withdrawal, chronic fatigue and lost enthusiasm for recreational activities, mood fluctuations, or a breakdown in communication. And, if someone is experiencing burnout or compassion fatigue, and they experience their partner as unsupportive, or not as supportive as they would like, this can lead to resentment.

Burnout can usually be resolved with a change in schedule, change in job, or time away from work. But compassion fatigue often requires a significant change in lifestyle and/or profession to help you get back to a state of equilibrium.

Not sure if you are burned-out? Here are a few statements to consider to better understand your risk for or experience of burnout. Count how many of the following statements resonate with you. The greater number of items you endorse, the more likely it is you are experiencing burnout.

- I experience frequent difficulties concentrating or sustaining attention on my work.

- I have noticed a decline in my problem-solving abilities and overall cognitive flexibility.

- I frequently feel emotionally exhausted, even after a full night of sleep.

- I struggle to find joy or satisfaction in my work or personal life.

- I have a hard time falling asleep or staying asleep.

- I do not feel refreshed, even after a good night's sleep.

- I experience persistent headaches, stomachaches, or muscle tension.

- I have noticed either an increase or decrease in my appetite.

- I have a hard time motivating myself to start or complete tasks.

- I feel detached or cynical about my work, colleagues, or industry.
- I am putting in consistent effort, but notice a drop in my overall productivity.
- I am struggling to meet deadlines that were once manageable.
- My personal and/or professional relationships feel strained.
- I feel isolated and have withdrawn from social activities.
- I have less time for self-care practices, like exercise, hobbies, or relaxation.
- I find myself neglecting my own needs in favor of work-related demands.
- I feel less competent at work and a decreased sense of accomplishment.
- I doubt the value and significance of my work.
- I've noticed more frequent or more intense mood swings, ranging from irritability to sadness, without an obvious cause.
- I find it difficult to switch off from work-related thoughts during my personal time.
- My emotional responses are often disproportionate to the situation.
- My work is dominating my life, and I find it difficult to establish balance.
- I question the meaning and purpose of my work and its impact on my life.
- I feel a lack of fulfillment or significance in my professional endeavors.
- I feel a lack of control over my life or work.
- I feel hopeless in some situations.

- I constantly feel fatigued and without enough energy to perform my daily tasks.

- I find it challenging to muster energy for activities I once enjoyed, including sex.

- I am making more errors in my work, or overlooking details I would typically catch.

- I have received feedback about the decreased quality of my work.

- I have noticed hesitation or indecisiveness in my decision-making processes.

- I am more likely to avoid making decisions altogether.

- I feel a sense of time pressure, as if there is never enough time to complete my to-do list.

- I frequently lose track of time, and find it challenging to prioritize and manage my schedule.

- I feel less consciously attuned to my mental health and well-being.

- I have sought professional help to address my concerns about my mental or physical well-being.

- When reflecting on my career and personal achievements, I struggle to find a sense of satisfaction.

- I am dismissive of my successes, and attribute them to external factors instead of my efforts.

- When I think about my professional future, I feel pessimistic.

- I have considered alternative professional paths or lifestyle strategies as a way to improve my well-being.

I'm a Stay-at-Home Parent, I Can't Be Burned-Out

Yes, you can. Being a stay-at-home parent, or domestic engineer, is work. Hard work. Often self-depriving work. And being a parent, especially the primary parent—which a stay-at-home parent often is—can add an extra element to burnout. The demands of your kids are never-ending, even in quiet moments. For many parents, the mental load you carry is a constantly running narrative of everything you have to remember, have to *remember* to remember, have to delegate, follow up on, purchase, wash and dry, put away, get ready, and so the list goes on.

On top of that, primary parents or parents who are nursing can feel "touched out"—another way parents often feel when burned-out. To be touched out means your body is overstimulated from all of the physical touch demands being put on you by children who need you—need to touch you, be seen by you, be heard by you, and be bathed, dressed, fed, and hugged by you. Countless parents, especially mothers, live in shame because they feel they are not doing enough, and feel buried by the physical and emotional demands of parenting, while their bodies are giving out from fatigue and exhaustion.

Frequently a surprise for new parents, the experience of being touched out can be a real impediment to sexual desire or arousal. Touch in this context becomes encoded with a sense of obligation, and a feeling that your body is not really your own. Not only are you likely exhausted, but the physical experience of so much one-sided attunement can implicitly render you emotionally drained, too. Self-care becomes a thing of the past, if it was ever a well-established practice to begin with, and mothers often become a living version of *The Giving Tree*,[6] being in a near constant state of deprivation without adequate restoration. Perhaps you're lucky and have had enough support from others that your self-care routine has been on point since having kids. That is not the case for many parents, and the effects can be long reaching. Taking space for yourself, and being supported in that effort, is the best way to prevent or recover from feeling touched out.

In the brilliant book *Touched Out: Motherhood, Misogyny, Consent, and Control*,[7] Amanda Montei highlights the many demands of motherhood, and writes, "There's the existential and personal upheaval, the difficulty of tracking where the parent's body ends and the baby begins." She continues that the experience of motherhood is often paired with a notable social contract. Self-sacrifice in service of your home is the path of morality and social standing. However, the cost of being socially acceptable is often being and feeling desexualized and exhausted. The price of being a "good" mother is pleasure, and for many women, their rest, pleasure, and sexuality are deprioritized and relegated to one of the duties of being a good partner. Imagine one more person who needs you for their pleasure or well-being, without consideration and mutual support. Some of you reading this won't have to imagine; you know this feeling well and being touched out is not just about the kids but also your partner's bids for your body that feel overwhelmingly about *their* pleasure, and without care for the state of your rest or arousal.

Kate Manne coined the term "human giver" in her book *Down Girl: The Logic of Misogyny*[8] to denote the differences between how men and women are socialized in general, and especially about care tasks. She explains a hallmark feature of systemic misogyny is that men are often socialized to be human *beings*, whereas women are socialized to be human *givers*, highlighting how men are expected to be centered in their family lives and society, while women are expected to be in service of those men.

What does this have to do with burnout and desire? A lot. Prolific sex researcher Emily Nagoski and her sister Amelia Nagoski dove deep into the double standards between men and women* with regard to stress and burnout in their book *Burnout: The Secret to Unlocking the Stress Cycle*.[9] The Nagoski sisters elaborate on the phenomenon, calling it "human giver syndrome," and outlining the many implications and disparities for women consistently being conditioned to put everyone before themselves. Enter all of the common sayings about how you have to put your own oxygen mask on first, and can't draw water from an empty well.

There is truth to these sayings in that you cannot expect to be in one-sided dynamics, whether at work, in a partnership, as a parent, or with friends, without time for restoration and some level of reciprocity from the adult relationships in your life, without expecting your vitality to plummet. Countless researchers point to the reality that when our bodies are under-resourced, they begin to shut down. The physician Gabor Maté wrote a whole book dedicated to the idea that the body demonstrates symptoms of disease as a way of saying no when we do not have the ability to change our life circumstances in the face of stress, or do not exercise adequate boundaries with our time and in our relationships.[10]

Finding Balance

If you're feeling a lack of desire, and if this chapter resonates for you, it may be time to have an honest conversation with yourself (and your partner) about how to work toward a more sustainable balance. Take an honest inventory of your daily workload and to-do list. Where (if anywhere) can you do less? Can you and your partner (if

---

* The research does not adequately address the impact of stress on folks who identity outside the gender binary.

you have one) create a new, sustainable approach to navigating the needs of your unit, reciprocally? Can you create or lean on friends or family with a system of support where you barter your strengths in exchange for some support from them? For example, if you're really good with meal prep, perhaps you offer your friend or neighbor a week's worth of prepped meals in exchange for them watching your kids on a Saturday, so you can read, go to the gym, sleep, or do whatever helps you find some restoration. Offer something that is relatively easy for you to manage in exchange for something that is relatively easy for another.

CASE STUDY

Anne doesn't have children, but she noted one of the things that really took it out of both her and partner was cleaning up after their dog in the yard. One of their neighbor's kids loved their dog, and was looking for a part-time job. Anne spoke with the preteen's parents, and with their approval, she offered him a part-time job to come over twice each week to play with the dog and clean up its waste. It cost her only twenty-five dollars each week, and in exchange her dog was being exercised and entertained, the yard was free of excrement, and she got four hours back in her week, enough time to do some yoga, watch a little TV, and take a nice bath. Within a month, she was feeling much better and was surprised by how quickly she started to feel more desire.

Anne and her partner had run out of ideas about how to get back some extra time in their lives. Used to relying just on each other to find much-needed respite, they were at a loss on how to make time for restoration. By talking about their options, they realized that offloading one of their time-consuming tasks each week and spending a little money would be a manageable solution for them.

Curating balance is an active process and may feel like it takes more energy than you have to give at the moment, complicating your ability to move beyond this point of exhaustion into a sense of embodied vitality. What would it take? If you ruled the universe and could have everything exactly as it should be, what would be different in your life that would give you space to feel more alive and energized?

Pleasure Points

- Burnout is a thief of energy and erotic potential, and it can affect your life beyond the workplace.

- Parents can experience burnout from the demands of their often unpaid domestic and emotional labor, and can feel touched out from the physical touch demands of parenting, further complicating their relationship with desire.

- The path to balance often requires energy that is difficult to mine, and getting support from coworkers, friends, family, and your partner is essential in reestablishing a more sustainable lifestyle.

- It can be difficult to recognize the subtle signs of burnout, such as cynicism at work, feeling like your efforts do not matter, and feeling constantly exhausted and/or less competent, especially if your achievements and work ethic are being praised or you're operating in survival mode.

Pleasure Reflections

- How has your relationship with work changed over the years? How would you describe your level of satisfaction with your workload, achievements, and balance?

- Are you experiencing any of the other physical symptoms related to stress, such as headaches, stomach problems, muscle tension, or sleep disruption? How do these symptoms affect your relationship with desire?

- If you are a parent, or in any caregiving role, do you feel touched out or physically overstimulated by the physical contact of care tasks? If so, how might that play a role in how readily you feel desire?

- If you resonated with anything in this chapter, what steps might you take to begin to shift your day-to-day balance? What obstacles, if any, might prevent you from making changes?

Chapter 5

Am I Numb?

A question I often ask clients when they are struggling with desire or lack of sexual pleasure is, "How present are you?" The response is mixed, but a few common themes emerge. Some people know right off the bat that they are not *really* present or mindful, and they move through the day on autopilot. Some respond with assurances about all the meditation they do—or *should* do, but don't have the time for. And some look perplexed and ask what it even means to "be present." It's a fair question since there is so much content floating around about mindfulness and presence and embodiment, but what those terms mean in daily life can be confusing. Others assert they are *very* present and feel *super* connected to the here and now. No matter where you're starting, you can always build your relationship with pleasure and presence.

The second question I generally ask is, "Can you tell me about your embodiment practice?" Embodiment is a term used to explore the way in which people live through and are aware of the sensory experiences of their bodies. This question usually evokes even more curiosity and uncertainty than the first. It is easy to disconnect from your body, as Western society does not encourage a lot of embodiment practice. The drive to get by with our overloaded schedules and commitments can legitimately make it difficult to slow down enough to be present, conscious, or mindful in our bodies.

Being present 24-7 is neither possible nor ideal; it takes up a lot of mental energy, and we know the brain is all about conserving energy and resources. We could not function if we were tuned in to every one of our senses every moment of every day. Having moments of less presence allows us to function. It would be challenging to get anything done if all you did was attune to the sensations in your body as they were happening. However, not spending enough time in, or intention on, the present can lead people to become less sensitive to their thoughts, emotions, senses, bodily cues, and behavior. Living chronically in this state can make you feel numb.

Some people may experience feeling numb when they are burned-out, and others may feel numb but do not relate to burnout. Feeling numb can happen for myriad reasons. In this chapter, I'll consider numbness primarily as a response to any kind of chronic disconnection with your body or emotions. Some may also consider this to be a functional freeze state (a survival response in which a person becomes "frozen" when confronted with real or perceived danger) or a functional collapse state (a decrease or shutdown of their body's typical level of functioning, which can include extreme fatigue, difficulty with simple everyday tasks, feelings of helplessness, difficulties with concentration or memory, or impaired decision-making). Trauma, dissociation, depression, substance use, addiction, and burnout can all contribute.

Emotional Numbness

If you experience a lack of emotion or a reduced level of emotional responsiveness to situations that would normally evoke a response for you, you may be emotionally numb. Perhaps you feel flat or as though your emotions have little range or movement. It can be difficult to connect with your emotions, express your feelings, notice them in your body, or react to situations that would typically evoke joy, happiness, sadness, or distress. For example, imagine you just received the good news that your best friend is coming to visit. You haven't seen her in a long time and you miss her terribly. But you're surprised to discover that you don't really feel anything. You want to be excited and cognitively you are, but you don't *feel* any enthusiasm.

Physical Numbness

Physical numbness can be understood from a lack of sensation in your body or reduced sensitivity to sensory data in various parts of the body. Physical injuries, nerve damage, poor circulation, or some medical conditions can render you less aware of sensation in the body. Some physical numbness is transient, whereas some may be chronic due to medical conditions or injuries. Some people feel "numbness" on their genitals and wonder if it's in response to their overuse of a vibrator. Vibrators do not cause permanent numbness or desensitization of your genitals, and for the approximate 16.5 percent of vulva owners who reported genital numbness after vibrator use, sensation generally returned after variations in feeling were introduced or use of a vibrator stopped for a period of time.[1]

Numbness may not mean that you feel nothing. You may in fact feel tingling or a "pins and needles" sensation instead of loss of any feeling. Perhaps parts of your body react as if they are on mute when processing sensory information with a reduced sensitivity to pleasure or pain. Some sexual trauma survivors report genital numbness, because of the trauma. For some, that can be rooted in physical damage to the vulva, vagina, or clitoris. Others do not bear sustained physical injury, and instead often experience numbness in their genitals as a result of underdeveloped communication between the genitals and the somatosensory part of the brain (this is the part of the brain responsible for interpreting sensation in various body parts). Dissociation during trauma, especially if the sexual trauma was chronic over time and occurred early in life, can interrupt these mind–body communications, leaving some survivors with a lack of perceptible sensation.

Relational Numbness

Having difficulty feeling anything when you're around others, or struggling to form or maintain emotional connections, can be an indication of relational numbness. This could be rooted in attachment concerns, fear of vulnerability, or a history of trauma, and may limit your ability to feel connected with another person. You may feel less trusting or more distant, while also not especially reactive about it.

Sexual Numbness

Having a limited, reduced, or absent ability to experience sexual pleasure or arousal can be understood as sexual numbness. This may manifest as having a diminished interest in sex, challenges with arousal, or a hard time having an orgasm.

There are many factors that may underlie and reinforce a feeling of being numb. Here are some of the most common.

- A history of trauma (physical, emotional, sexual, relational, spiritual, financial, racial, etc.)
- Symptoms of post-traumatic stress

- Burnout or chronic stress
- Depression, anxiety, or other mood disorders
- Dissociation
- Grief and loss
- Witnessing violence, accidents, or a natural disaster
- Conflict or betrayal in a relationship
- Social isolation and loneliness
- Professional dissatisfaction, unemployment, or underemployment
- Drug or alcohol abuse, addiction or withdrawal
- Compulsive behavior
- Persistent health concerns
- Side effects of medication
- Disordered eating
- Poor body image or body dysphoria
- Alexithymia (difficulty identifying and naming emotions, discerning between emotions, and communicating them to others)
- Chronic busyness or overfunctioning
- History of pain during sex

Am I Numbing Out?

In some instances, people unconsciously stay in a cycle of avoiding uncomfortable things by numbing out as a coping mechanism. It's not always intentional, but it may give you some space from difficult emotions, creating a buffer and self-protection to manage overstimulation, avoid triggers related to previous trauma, or maintain a sense of self-control. What can be an adaptive short-term coping mechanism to maintain psychological equilibrium can lead to chronic feelings of numbness or being perpetually checked out or on autopilot. Used in the long term, this approach to managing distress can interfere with personal mindfulness, growth, maturity, authenticity, connection, and pleasure.

A common form of numbing out is compulsive behavior or addiction. Ritualized behavior can become rhythmic, as its predictability prompts a neurochemical experience that does not require much presence, while also shifting your emotional or physiological states. Many substances and some behaviors associated with process (behavioral) addictions activate the reward center in the brain, causing the release of dopamine. However, chronic participation in the ritual can make this natural release of dopamine less effective in changing one's mood or state. Addiction can desensitize a person's baseline levels of pleasure and reward, leading to neuroadaptation (tolerance) and rendering it more difficult to experience joy or pleasure in activities that are not part of the addictive ritual without more dopamine.[2]

When the same stimulus fails to evoke the desired reaction due to repeated use, it can lead to tolerance, and a desire for increasing amounts of the same stimulus to reach the desired effect. Tolerance can impact neural circuits and structural changes in areas of the brain connected to emotional processing and regulation, decision-making abilities, and impulse control.[3] If those areas are impacted, a person's emotional responsiveness may also change, leading to feelings of numbness or under-responsiveness. A common complaint for folks in early recovery from addiction is that nothing is fun, or they feel like they are just going through the motions. This is because their brain may be used to processing stimulation at a very high level, so it can take a while for it to recalibrate to less intense stimuli. Sometimes, the brain is permanently affected.

Not sure if you're numbing out? Here are a few ways to tell.

- You feel emotionally flat or have a hard time noticing a range of emotions.

- You catch yourself frequently daydreaming, spacing out, feeling disconnected from the current moment.

- Your everyday tasks or activities get completed without much conscious awareness or thought—you're on autopilot.

- You avoid conversations or situations that you expect will be laden with strong emotions.

- You are not clear about how you feel in any given moment or can't identify specific emotions from others.

- You generally feel checked out, indifferent, or apathetic toward things in which you once found pleasure or joy.

- You love the escape and rely on substances, gaming, social media, TV/movies, food-related behaviors, work, and so on, to decompress or reset.

- You are less motivated to engage in social activities, less interested in catching up with people, or avoid anything beyond a superficial connection.

- You may be stuck in a rut or a boring routine, unconsciously avoiding novel situations, as novelty often comes with emotional charge.

- You may fixate on anything that gives you a sense of control, such as perfectionist behavior, rigid adherence to rules, or structure, as predictability minimizes the likelihood of being caught off guard by unanticipated emotions.

Am I Numb or Dissociated?

Dissociation, a process in which someone feels disconnected from their thoughts, feelings, sensations, or surroundings, often in a surreal way, shares many features with numbness. It can be helpful to think about numbness and dissociation as related feelings on a continuum. Both are a type of disconnection. Both limit your ability to embrace or experience life in a meaningful way. While numbness often leaves you feeling muted, flat, or having a one-dimensional experience of a situation, dissociation often feels surreal, as if you are observing yourself from a distance (depersonalization) or as if your surroundings are distorted or not real (derealization).[4]

A disconnection between mind and body can leave someone who has dissociated with pockets of time they cannot recall, or feeling as though they've been in a dreamlike state. They can struggle to remember parts or all of the dissociated moments as some elements of memory can be impacted in a dissociated state.[5] Dissociation often leads to disconnection from yourself, your identity, your body, and in some severe cases, even reality.

Because dissociation can feel so surreal, it can be tricky to tell when you're experiencing it. Here are key indicators that you may be experiencing dissociation.

- Losing time, forgetting parts of or whole events
- Forgetting parts of or all conversations you had while in a dissociative state
- Feeling like you're not really where you are
- Feeling as though you're watching yourself from above or at a distance
- Having a hard time focusing or feeling foggy
- Not being able to recognize yourself in the mirror

- Feeling like you're going through the motions of a given activity
- Feeling like what's happening to you is happening to someone else
- Feeling like your emotions are not really yours
- Feeling disconnected from specific body parts or your whole body
- Being spatially disoriented, or getting lost even when you're familiar with the environment
- Feeling unable to track or express your feelings
- Perceptual changes, such as having tunnel vision or seeing distorted colors, or hearing sounds as muted or amplified
- Seeming unresponsive or indifferent to an experience that would otherwise warrant a reaction
- Avoiding people, places, or things that remind you of traumatic or difficult events
- Having difficulty making decisions, or being impulsive in your decision-making

Chronic numbness and dissociation can become a feedback loop whereby you live in a low-grade state of being less present, and so do not develop adequate coping skills to effectively regulate intense emotions. Then, when you feel those emotions, they may trigger a more dissociated state and rupture the conscious connection between mind and body, which can leave you feeling muted, disconnected from yourself or others, confused, foggy, or like you are observing your life instead of truly living it.

Both numbness and dissociation can make you feel disembodied, a key barrier to feeling pleasure. To be embodied means to be in a state of awareness, connection, and presence, in the here and now, in your own body. It means that you can actively feel and experience physical sensations, emotions, and movements in your body. Also referred to as the "soma," the body contains valuable information about the state of your well-being or distress. Staying present with that information helps us better understand and protect ourselves from threat, as well as expand our potential for pleasure. So, when someone is feeling disembodied, they lose connection to that valuable information, and therefore to a part of themselves. Disconnecting from one's own somatic cues can restrict a relationship with the self and reduce a sense of physical presence. Embodiment and disembodiment exist on a continuum and we move back and forth along it. Stress and traumatic experiences push us toward disembodiment while coping strategies or supports push us back to embodiment.

CASE STUDY

Jimena started sex therapy after years of feeling frustrated with her inability to have an orgasm. When she first started having partnered sex with her boyfriend in college she had no problem having orgasms. However, shortly after graduating college, she learned that he had been having an emotional and sexual affair with her best friend. Jimena's best friend was dating her boyfriend's best friend, and all this time, she had thought they were the ideal friend group. They all hung out together just about every weekend, and Jimena couldn't figure out when her boyfriend and best friend had had time to have an affair. She was devastated, and both couples *and* both sets of best friends broke up. Overnight, Jimena lost her two closest people and a built-in social group. She took a few months to get her bearings and then moved to a new city where she eventually started dating again.

Age twenty-four, Jimena was ready for love again. But she was also busy with a new job, trying to make new friends, and feeling wary of everyone. Most of the men she dated were quick to make things sexual, which left her feeling discouraged about prospects for a relationship with a man her age. She was fine with casual sex and actually thought it might be better for her, to avoid getting her heart broken again. That, she couldn't handle. However, Jimena never had sex that felt fulfilling. It's not that she was sexually incompatible with the majority of partners, although that was the case for some; she just didn't feel much during sex anymore. She had a good enough time, but couldn't reach orgasm. At the time, she chalked it up to casual dating, and thought she might just be someone who needs an emotional connection to come.

Four years later, Jimena had just completed grad school and got a new job. She and some friends were out celebrating, and she met a man who would quickly become important to her. Jimena felt different about him, she felt safe; she even felt safe introducing him to her friends. He knew about the infidelity she'd experienced and took great care to assure her of his dedication to her and their relationship. He was attentive and focused on her pleasure. She trusted him implicitly. But even after a year, she could not have an orgasm with him. Beyond that, during sex, Jimena often felt little to no sensation. It felt good, or at least she told herself it did, but she couldn't really *feel* any sensation. She felt like she was watching herself have sex from across the room.

After some time, she felt bad and didn't want to disappoint him by not having an orgasm. Jimena was worried that if he didn't think their sex life was good enough, he might be tempted to cheat. There it was. She was still harboring fear about her safety in the relationship and wondered if he would cheat on her eventually, too. She didn't consciously believe he would, but she didn't believe her ex would have, either. So, how could she be sure? Jimena's head was spinning and she felt disconnected from her body as a result of the betrayal. Perhaps this was part of why she couldn't orgasm?

For many people, the experience of pleasure and especially orgasm feels incredibly vulnerable. One has to surrender to a feeling that is out of your control. The French refer to an orgasm as "la petite mort,"[6] or the little death, because during an orgasm some people report feeling an alteration of consciousness or state of transcendence. Resembling a temporary release of the ordinary, this step into ecstasy can feel so powerfully unyielding and out of control that it feels like a small, metaphorical death. It's wonderful if you feel safe enough to let go and flurry around in such untethered bliss. But without safety, that surrender can feel too dangerous, and may be perceived as a threat against which protection is needed.

How Is This Affecting My Desire?

When you have to use the bathroom, you generally know because you can feel the internal cue that your bladder is full. You know you're hungry when you feel pangs in your stomach, bridging your awareness to your need to eat. This is interoception, the perception of internal cues. Interoception also alerts us to the physiological sensations of arousal, such as an increased heart rate and genital sensation, and helps you deduce subjective desire. When you experience numbness, dissociation, or other forms of disembodiment, sensory data is limited or not available due to interrupted or underdeveloped interoception. If you are struggling to be attuned to your body and its cues, there may not be enough sensory information communicated between the brain and body to signal pleasure.

This is especially the case for childhood sexual trauma survivors, who may have experienced dissociation during or following the abuse. Consider this metaphor: In order to build a road between two cities, a path needs to be cleared of trees, bushes, and other obstructions, then leveled before the cement can be poured and a freeway established. Without that completed, people going to and from each city may have to take indirect routes, or may not even know how to get there at all. When abuse happens during periods of critical brain development, dissociation prevents the road (neuropathways) from properly developing. The good news is this can change with focused interoceptive skill building and mindfulness.

Pain During Sex and Avoidance

A special note to consider about numbing out is that it may be in response to sexual pain. Pain during penetration can leave people feeling confused, angry, helpless, powerless, and at odds with themselves, and can lead to fear during future sexual activities. For some, the fear of future painful sex experiences can result in a cycle of catastrophizing, which can cause more fear—and then bracing, tension, or vigilance in their bodies and more pain. For many, avoiding sex and anything that reminds them of sex becomes the only way to detach from the reality of the depression or wariness caused by both the pain they are enduring and the ramifications of it in their lives.[7] Numbing out, or even feelings of disgust, may arise as a psychological barrier to the anticipation of pain. Some researchers suggest that sexual disgust (disgust about some or all things sexual) may create a tendency of pain during sex for some people.[8] While for others, pain may result in disgust as a response to the idea or practice of sex. Avoidance or numbing out becomes a practice to block out one's awareness of either pain or disgust in these instances.

The path back to pleasure starts with a willingness to feel. If you've been feeling numb or dissociated for a while, especially if numbing out has been your go-to coping strategy, coming back into your mind and body can feel intimidating or disorienting. In chapter 15, there is a step-by-step outline on how to get back in touch with your body.

Starting small is the best way to gradually reintroduce yourself to your bodily sensations, in a way that feels accessible and tolerable. Perhaps taking a few minutes a day to dance to music can help you stay present, without judgment, with the way your body moves and undulates to various sounds. Don't worry about what you look like. Stay curious about how you feel, what you see around you, the music you hear, and so on. Staying connected to your senses in small doses can help bring you back into your body, but if you feel flooded (overwhelmed by your emotions or sensations), it's OK to shift your attention to something external. Can you count the tiles on the floor, the number of flowers outside the window, or name all of the books with an orange cover on your bookshelf? When you feel more regulated, perhaps take another small dose of internal curiosity, repeating the pattern of observing what is internal and then what is external.

Pleasure Points

- Changes in sexual desire can indicate a bigger problem, such as burnout or unresolved trauma, or a lack of presence or embodiment.

- Numbness and dissociation are similar in many ways, but dissociation represents a great rupture in one's self-perception, identity, and sometimes reality.

- Numbing out can be a way people avoid pain or discomfort, whether physical or emotional.

- Childhood sexual abuse survivors may struggle with numbness during sex, as dissociation from the childhood trauma may have limited the amount of sensory data that the brain perceives from the genitals.

- Interoception, the perceptions of internal stimuli or physiological cues in your body, is a key ingredient in being present.

- Sexual pain can become a precursor to disembodiment, during sex or otherwise, and can lead to avoidance of desire or participation in sexual activities.

Pleasure Reflections

- As you reflect on feeling numb, dissociated, or not fully in your body, ask yourself what you may not want to be feeling. Are there realities in your life that, when faced consciously, bring up dysregulating or confusing emotions?

- In what ways might you be feeling numb or less connected to yourself? What factors contribute to this feeling?

- Have you ever felt dissociation? What signs or symptoms can you recall? Has it ever affected your sexual pleasure?

Chapter 6

Am I Angry or Bitter?

In exploring changes in libido, a common dismissive complaint from some partners is that their partner is "just angry and bitter" about an ongoing conflict, and "that's why they don't want to have sex." They may not be wrong, though their dismissiveness about lingering anger surely does not help to solve the problem of desire.

Anger is a protective emotion. When you feel anger, it is a signal that you think something is unfair or unjust, or that you feel disrespected in some way. Anger stands out from the rest of our emotions as a powerful player, capable of shaping the arousal of our nervous system, and consequently, our sexual arousal. Many people who come to sex therapy looking to reconnect with desire don't immediately understand the connection their anger has to their libido (or lack thereof). After some careful unpacking, it is often clear unresolved anger or resentment remains a barrier.

Anger, or rather the destructive expression of anger, gets a bad rap. You may be surprised to hear that anger is invaluable once you know how to recognize it and communicate it effectively. It is a teacher, a guide, a wisdom that all of us are born with as a means of self-protection. Anger is a natural fight-or-flight response to real or perceived threats to our sense of self or to violations of our personal boundaries. It signals that a line has been crossed, alerting us that something is not OK. And it is necessary in healthy relationships. Anger expressed in prosocial and productive ways compels assertiveness, appropriate boundary-setting, and sets the stage for your needs and values to be acknowledged and respected.

The discomfort felt in a state of anger or resentment is fuel to remedy situations that threaten your survival or well-being. Without anger, you may not take action to right the situation. Anger and resentment give way to self-advocacy and the restoration of power and justice. Yet, when suppressed, anger and resentment can become heavy, sedentary emotions that block creativity, eros, and connection.

It's no surprise that if your romantic or sexual relationship is riddled with implicit power struggles or imbalances, anger and resentment are familiar emotional states. This is your body's way of letting you know it's time to rebalance the scales of fairness and integrity. In dating, sexual, and romantic relationships, power imbalances (especially those that remain unexplored or unresolved) can lead to tremendous anger in the relationships, significantly impacting desire. When a partner consistently exerts control or dominance, or when multiple partners do so over time, resentment and helplessness may ensue. This dynamic is often observed in heterosexual relationships in which one or both partners endorse men to have more power or authority. In these settings, it is common for women to feel undervalued, stifled, or oppressed. A lack of mutual respect and equitable problem-solving can disrupt connection, felt safety, and trust. Who wants to have sex then?

Anger is also a beacon of autonomy, providing a crucial sign that we feel enveloped by external pressures or confronted with manipulation. Anger shields us from withering in inertia and fortifies our resolve against unwanted influences or participation in our own neglect. When we feel overlooked, anger draws our awareness to the gaping disparity so we can advocate for our own fulfillment. It can also serve as a protection against vulnerability or hurt. Long-term resentment is often a shield against ongoing disappointment, shame, disconnection, or loneliness. It is usually easier to stay angry or resentful than to really sit with the difficult and often painfully powerless feelings of being disappointed or let down repeatedly—a likely outcome when there is inadequate repair or restoration in interpersonal relationships.

It is beneficial for the health of a relationship for you and your partner to feel and effectively communicate your anger with each other. Doing so communicates a desire to stay in the relationship and gives you a roadmap to address the felt imbalances so you can get back to a place of equanimity.

CASE STUDY

"My boyfriend doesn't initiate sex with me, ever!" Nia was furious in her first session. She continued that he often said how attracted to her he was, and he complained frequently that they were not having enough sex. But he rarely initiated sex. Nia was tired of being the person to always initiate. She begged him to initiate more—not even all the time, just more! He said he would, but he didn't. She brought it up again and told him how important it was to her that they both initiate sex, because she wasn't turned on by always having to get things going. He deflected her bid and said he was used to other women initiating sex in his previous relationships. They had been together for nearly five years, and during the first year of their relationship, Nia recalled a more even balance in their invitations with one another. She told her boyfriend that she was "only matching his energy" from now on, meaning that if he initiated sex one time, she would initiate it the next. But she would not initiate first. He had to do it. They didn't have sex for nearly a year. Nia was furious and resentful, nursing feelings of powerlessness and hurt.

In later sessions, Nia declared she was ready to end the relationship, but didn't want to give up on what she thought was otherwise an incredible relationship. But he needed to show up differently, she said, so she bought him some books that would help strengthen their relationship and communication skills, and even got some board games for couples to deepen their intimacy. She asked him to take some initiative, plan some dates, bring some romance into their life, but he didn't. He was inert and could not offer a substantive explanation for his lack of effort, beyond that he wasn't used to being asked to do these things prior to this relationship and was doing his best to change with her requests. This was infuriating to Nia, who did not believe he was really invested in change. When she told him she wanted to end the relationship, he was shocked and promised to do anything she asked. He got it now, or so he said. But he didn't. And she was tired of carrying their relationship. She wanted a partner who met her needs or could at least communicate with her if he couldn't show up. Why couldn't he see how important this was to her? She brought it up again and he said he would, but his words never materialized into action. Over the course of several therapy sessions, she decided she couldn't wait any longer, and she ended the relationship.

Again, he was tearful and promised to prioritize her needs, and convinced her to try again. He went to therapy, read the books, and agreed to start initiating sex. But he didn't. After much conversation, a deal was begrudgingly brokered: She would set up the volley so her boyfriend could close, and they could both agree that he had been the one to initiate sex. She would tell him she was horny and he could interpret that as a guaranteed yes to sex if he made a move to kiss her or lead her to the bedroom. After all this time, he was able to articulate that he was nervous he'd get rejected and this was the reason he didn't initiate.

Yet she admitted in therapy that when they finally had sex, she wasn't even turned on. Her desire was zapped. In fact, she noticed that she was having different sensory experiences—she hated the way he smelled and felt disgusted by his touch. She was so angry at him that her body was repulsed at the idea of being sexually close, even though that is what she'd wanted for the longest time. She felt lost and completely detached from her sexuality and her partner. When he did bring up sex, she got annoyed and angry. She wanted to respond with enthusiasm, but she was spent. All she could feel in her body was the cold hard deadness of resentment.

Anger and Desire

Stress hormones—adrenaline and cortisol—surge in the body as the sympathetic nervous system (the activation of fight-or-flight reactions) responds to anger. These hormones prepare the body for action, redirecting resources away from any nonessential survival functions, including sexual arousal. The signs of this sympathetic nervous system arousal often include an increased heart rate, heightened alertness, and muscle tension. It's hardly surprising that the response that primes the body for combat, however real or imagined, impedes connection and acts as a formidable barrier to the relaxation and receptivity necessary for a satisfying sexual experience. A spark of anger may flood your sympathetic nervous system with energy, while keeping you from feeling relaxed enough to connect to any sustainable desire.

You may be thinking: *But I get turned on when I'm angry!* Some people do, and the release of oxytocin that follows intimate contact and orgasm can help to reduce the experience of stress in the body. In other words, oxytocin reduces the level of cortisol,[1] and for some people, anger can be felt in the body like other upregulating emotions—anxiety, fear, and even excitement. A sympathetically aroused nervous system can amplify sexual arousal. In fact, this is part of the appeal for some kink and fetish play—but more on that later.

Internalized anger or resentment, on the other hand, can feel like a slow burn, with their roots tangled in unresolved grievances. A perpetual state of resentment can become a silent saboteur. With a persistent grip, resentment can keep the body in a chronic state of (often low-level) stress, humming with sympathetic arousal, and limiting the ability of the parasympathetic nervous system (our sensations of relaxation and calm) to fully assert its restful influence. Too much cortisol in the body can feel exhausting.

Imagine you have one foot on the gas and one foot on the brake at the same time—the car will exhaust the gas in the tank (or the charge on the battery), but it won't go anywhere. This is the effect of chronic resentment on your libido. Your body struggles to shift into the receptive or relaxed state that sexual arousal requires. It can be difficult to be vulnerable without fear when your body is in a chronic state of low-level fight-or-flight due to ongoing resentments. And if you are harboring resentment toward your partner, it makes perfect sense that your body would not feel safe enough to experience desire with that person. An unpopular truth is that this can be a catalyst for extra-relational affairs.[2] Desire is hard to come by in a relationship shrouded by lingering resentment.

Not only that but unresolved anger and resentment can have destructive effects on your body image and self-esteem. Remember that anger can signal injustice, disrespect, or feeling devalued, which triggers a core somatic response of powerlessness or helplessness. This is why the sympathetic nervous system gets activated—it gives a boost of power to counterbalance the somatic experience of having none. If, over time, you continue to feel helpless and powerless to change your circumstances, it can shift the way you see yourself. A once-solid sense of autonomy can deteriorate into a distorted and internalized view of yourself as someone with no agency in your re-lationship, circumstance, or the world. As a result, your self-esteem can plummet, and you may believe you are undeserving or incapable of feeling in control. Your body image and confidence may become warped, leading you to believe you are undesired or undesirable. The manifestation of stress, tension, and a heightened state of hypervig-ilance can disrupt your mind/body harmony. This disconnect can re-sult in a belief that others view you as unworthy, as that incoherence is often internalized and felt as an inherent flaw.

Feeling powerless or helpless can also lead to self-neglect. Someone who has internalized mistreatment by others may feel disembodied, and can also neglect self-care, their physical appear-ance and well-being, style, and overall demeaner in a self-reinforcing vicious cycle, a pattern that does not leave room to cultivate or access sexual desire. Self-neglect can be an unconscious, albeit protective, attempt to dissuade the desire of another, by becoming less desirable to them, or it can be a form of self-advocacy in a form of protest.

Unsurprisingly, a low self-appraisal or negative self-perception can interfere with your ability to initiate sexual intimacy, by yourself or with a partner, due to the heightened feeling of inadequacy or fears of being nude (literally or figuratively) and vulnerable. These escalating insecurities and self-consciousness can exacerbate performance anxiety, fears of judgment, and ineffective communication about fantasies or desires. It can also limit boundary setting, reinforcing a negative self-appraisal and a fight-or-flight response, and separating you further and further from arousal (and bolstering even more resentments!).

Do I Have Permission to Be Angry?

People across the gender continuum can experience this disconnected state, and for those socialized as women, the effects of suppressed and unresolved anger or resentment can be amplified in their internalization, often manifesting a chronic stress, anxiety, depression, or psychosomatic symptoms like headaches, fatigue, or stomach issues, and in difficulty asserting and maintaining boundaries. Women are often expected to not only suppress anger, but to not experience it at all. From a young age, women are tasked with the responsibility of prioritizing harmony and avoiding conflict, to keep the peace and the power imbalance. Their authentic sense of self, autonomy, and expression of anger are often actively discouraged. Social expectations and biases rooted in patriarchal conditioning can reinforce suppression and internalization of anger, as well as shame for even experiencing it all, leading women to further shut down. Women who embrace their anger frequently face shame, ridicule, infantilization and/or retaliation and punishment, which unsurprisingly leads to more feelings of helplessness, powerlessness, and fear.[3]

Patriarchal narratives create a double bind for many women with regard to anger: They are denied the space to fully explore and address their anger (and therefore advocate for their personhood), while facing criticism for not self-advocating enough. Ever heard someone tell a woman to pick a better partner? Or just leave an abusive relationship? These are exemplary experiences of how women are often jostled into a position of perceiving themselves as having limited agency (and sometimes of actually *having* limited agency) and control over their lives, reluctant to assert boundaries or limits, or fear an inflamed sensitivity to judgment and social exclusion. These double-bind scenarios are often magnified in frequency and intensity for marginalized women, reflecting increased pressure on them to abandon themselves in service of systemic power structures.

HOW DOES THIS IMPACT YOUR SEX LIFE?

The political is personal, and the personal is political. Familial relationships are the first place where systemic power impacts our sense of self, autonomy, and respect in the world. Many children hear phrases from their parents such as, "Children are to be seen and not heard," sending a clear message that their voice and autonomy are not relevant and that they hold little to no power in the family system. How your caregivers addressed power in your early life was influenced by these greater social systems. In turn, this shapes your expectation of fairness, justice, and equality in your romantic and sexual relationships. If you are partnered with someone who does not respect your autonomy or does not respond sufficiently to your requests to repair a hurt you've expressed, you may receive the message that you don't matter, that you have no power, and that you have to subvert your needs in service of regulating your partner's emotions and keeping the peace in your relationship. That can fuel a level of shut-down resentment that is exhausting and debilitating, and the completely expected antithesis of sexual desire.

Because women are discouraged from being in touch with their anger, or shamed or punished when they do express it, many don't recognize the early indications of these emotions. Here are some common manifestations of anger and resentment. Which ones (if any) resonate with you?

- Ruminating about the perceived injustices in the relationship
- Comparing yourself to your partner, highlighting the perceived imbalances in power or accountability
- Fixating on your unmet needs and expectations in the relationship
- Feeling frustrated or annoyed over perceived neglect
- Feeling unappreciated
- Wanting your partner to understand and acknowledge your experience; working extra hard in an effort to be understood or validated
- Dwelling on instances where a partner's behavior has left you feeling distressed
- Ongoing doubts about your partner's commitment or intentions in the relationship
- Regular anger, irritability, or annoyance in response to your partner's needs or requests
- A growing awareness and discontent with the lack of perceived mutuality and reciprocity of effort or emotional support in the relationship

- Pulling away physically or emotionally (sharing less) as a protective measure
- Feeling a chronic negativity that underpins the relationships
- Feeling physiological symptoms of unease related to the relationship including, but not limited to, increased heart rate, palpitations, muscle tension, headaches, stomach discomfort or indigestion, shallow or rapid breathing, increased hypervigilance or startle response, fatigue and exhaustion, insomnia or difficulty staying asleep
- Feeling relieved when you have some space from your partner
- Feeling contempt or disgust when your partner wants something from you or tries to touch you
- Passive aggressive communication or behaviors become a frequent occurrence
- Avoiding having deep conversations; all of your conversations are superficial
- Decreasing interest in activities that might otherwise have been meaningful or enjoyable
- Exhibiting dismissive or dissatisfied body language
- Escalating conflicts or disagreements occur more readily and feel more personalized
- Seeking emotional support and validation from people other than your partner
- Engaging in small or big gestures that declare a sense of independence or autonomy (whether your partner knows about them or not)
- Excessively tracking or monitoring your partner's nonverbal communication and behavior to confirm the perceived grievances

So, Am I Angry and Bitter?

Probably. On some level. Even if what you're angry about is a lack of satisfying sex. It all builds when it is not resolved or repaired, and can lead to further disconnection from your erotic energy. As mentioned in chapter 2, disgust is a gatekeeping and boundary protecting emotion. So is anger. It's best to listen to it, give it credence and exploration, and work toward resolving it to reconnect with an affective state that allows you to feel safe, respected, and with autonomy. In many ways, anger can thwart desire. But if channeled into advocacy, it can ignite desire.

To get a handle on your anger, you can start by identifying the catalysts and triggers for it to help clarify some of the patterns that exist in your life and within your responses. Practicing grounding and progressive muscle relaxation exercises or breathwork can help to diffuse the escalation of anger in your body. Learning and practicing assertive communication with a trusted person (such as a friend, therapist, and so on) can help you with effective boundary setting and establishing clear expectations with others to avoid misunderstandings and possible conflicts.

Pleasure Points

- When anger is feared, misunderstood, or suppressed, its expression can be destructive. However, when understood and expressed in a constructive way, anger can serve as a teacher, guide, and blueprint for how to establish and maintain equity, justice, and interdependence in healthy relationships.

- Exploring and addressing anger and resentment in relationships is key in resolving power struggles, restoring balance, and ensuring all partners have a voice for self-advocacy.

- Chronic anger and resentment impact the nervous system, leaving the body in an acute or tempered state of fight or flight, releasing adrenaline and cortisol in the body, and decreasing desire.

- Women are especially at risk of resentment, given societal expectations around the suppression of their anger, prioritization of peacekeeping in relationships, expectations to subvert their own autonomy, and often retribution if they refuse.

Pleasure Reflections

- How do societal or gender-based expectations shape your relationship with anger—how you feel it and how you express it?

- Can you recall a positive instance when anger led you to be more assertive, resulting in your needs being met? How did you feel before, during, and after asserting yourself?

- How might unresolved anger or resentment be impacting your relationship with your body, self-care, or self-esteem?

- What are your earliest indications of resentment or anger? How have you typically communicated your experience, and with whom might you be able to seek support?

Part 2

What's Going On in My Relationships?

Every relationship has ups and downs, and even healthy relationships go through growing pains and chapters that feel off, but having unresolved or recurring ruptures (conflicts that create distance between you) can make it difficult to stay emotionally or sexually connected to a partner. It can be difficult to face the reality of what is or isn't feeling aligned in a relationship.

So much of what kept my sex life so stuck was an uncertainty about how much of what was shifting was *my* stuff, and how much was *our* stuff. This is true for most of the people I work with, because in relationships, what is individual often becomes relational. In my case, my partner and I both had personal baggage we brought to our dynamic, and we were both separately navigating uncharted territory in our growth. But even though our individual work was our own to sift though, there was leakage all over our relationship, so it became *our* stuff to process. We understood our dynamic differently and felt different levels of urgency about addressing it, which further complicated our waning desire.

So a loss of libido is not always a sign of relationship woes, but relationship woes can and often do get in the way of libido. The following are some of the most common relationship dynamics I see that thwart desire.

Am I Safe?

Feeling safe is a hallmark of desire and sexual pleasure. Even people who are turned on by risk or fear calculate how much they can tolerate to maximize pleasure, without being capsized by it. In fact, for many people, some element of fear accelerates desire and arousal, and this is often played out through exercises that may be considered taboo. Safety can be defined only by the absence of fear, but that doesn't always mean an absence of risk.

In thinking of safety, it's helpful to borrow from the world of Dialectical Behavior Therapy (DBT), which challenges black-and-white thinking and promotes living in the nuance or gray areas in life. It is important to recognize the trap of looking at people, places, or contexts as being either "safe" or "unsafe," as opposed to seeing safety on a spectrum. Seeing sex, relationships, or the world as safe or unsafe creates polarization and can lead to rigidity. Rarely are people or contexts either entirely safe or unsafe. There are degrees of safety and risk, and the variables are often changing, making one's appraisal of safety and risk an ongoing effort. How unsexy. And yet necessary.

In chapters 5 and 6, we established how the brain likes to conserve energy. That applies when assessing risk, too. So much so that many brains have a negativity bias, meaning they tend to look for danger cues more than safety cues to ensure they are likely to survive. It makes more sense for a mind trying to ensure our longevity to be more concerned about our demise than with the good stuff in life. Consider a worried parent telling a young child to look both ways before crossing the street. The young child is focused on seeing the neighbor's cute dog on the other side of the road, and not paying attention to their own safety amid the traffic. The concerned adult knows the risks, and is watching to make sure there are no cars or other dangers that may bar the child from getting across the street safely to play with the neighbor's dog. The parent is proactively looking for possible danger.

People tend to navigate around ambiguity by rushing to conclusions—to conserve energy—since ambiguity takes more energy to navigate than a simple conclusion. Rushing to judgment about what is safe (also known as a false positive) can leave us at greater risk of getting hurt, beyond what we've decided we can tolerate. And rushing to a conclusion that something is unsafe can thwart our ability to experience joy, pleasure, and growth. So, thinking of safety in binary terms doesn't help us maximize pleasure and minimize pain.

Moving beyond the black-and-white approach to safety to a continuum of safety and risk can help you shift to conceptualizing what feels *safer* or *safe enough* as you make decisions about your sexual and relational needs, and offer a better balance of pleasure and protection—and more access to your desire.

Defining Safe Enough

Because intimacy requires some level of vulnerability, there is always some risk of getting hurt. But it can be difficult to know what feels safe enough without first defining what feels unsafe for you. Pause here (or make a note for later) to write out a list of people, places, and contexts that you already know are immediate deal-breakers when it comes to feeling safe enough to be open to pleasure. For example, you might decide all lies are deal-breakers for you, or you might decide that little white lies about things like how much your partner likes the gift you've given them are OK. Or you might feel strongly that someone who is consistently late for dates is being disrespectful. No one can decide what feels safe enough for you, since people can assign different meanings to different behaviors. How do you know something is not safe enough for you? If this is the first time you're thinking about it, it's OK if you don't have clear answers. Beginning to pay attention is the starting point that can lead to empowerment. If you're not sure where to start, consider this chapter an invitation to begin exploring your own safety criteria. Take in some of the examples provided, and see how you feel. You can revisit your beliefs as you collect more information about how your body reacts in certain circumstances, and adjust your boundaries as you go.

Safety is subjective; what feels good for you may be someone else's red line. You may have a belief about what it means to be safe enough, and/or you may feel cues in your body that fear is on the rise. Some cognitive, emotional, and somatic cues that you are starting to feel less safe include the following.

- Increased heart rate
- Heightened sense of nervousness without a clear cause
- Constantly scanning your surroundings for potential threats (hypervigilance)
- Feeling uneasy, apprehensive, or suspicious of a situation or person

- Muscle tension or a tightening in your body
- Shallow or rapid breathing
- Feeling alone or disconnected from people around you
- Difficulty concentrating or staying focused
- Stomach discomfort or nausea
- A desire to avoid or escape a specific person, place, or situation
- Unexplained sensations of tingling or numbness, especially in your extremities
- Increased perspiration, even if you are not physically hot
- Feeling overwhelmed or overstimulated, or overly sensitive to noise, smell, or touch
- Feeling powerless or like you have little or no control in a situation
- Insomnia, or difficulty falling or staying asleep
- Feeling agitated or irritable
- Persistent negative thoughts

Which of these indicators are *your* body's way of alerting you that you feel less safe?

CASE STUDY

Brenda was eager to try new things sexually with her partner when they first got together. Her partner had a lot more sexual experience than she did and spent a lot of time watching porn. Specifically, he was turned on by cuckolding and wanted Brenda to join him in making this fantasy a reality. Brenda was open to the idea, but she wanted to take things slow because she had never imagined herself in such a position and wasn't sure how she felt about being sexual with another man.

Adding to her hesitance, Brenda's partner wanted her to take control of finding and arranging the other partner, so he could really feel cuckolded. Brenda had mixed feelings about taking this much initiative and was unsure about where to even start. Not used to playing with power dynamics or humiliation, Brenda was nervous about hurting her partner, as well as being able to find another person who was safe enough and would honor her requests for barrier use and STI testing before getting intimate. Brenda's partner was dismissive of her concerns and told her the chance of getting an STI was slim, but even if she did get one, he'd still love her, and it wouldn't be a problem for him. Brenda's heart rate increased and she felt sweaty, uneasy, suspicious, and nauseous. He'd still love *her*? She was baffled that he was not taking her concerns seriously and instead tried to reassure her that he would still desire her! What about how she felt? What she desired? In that moment, she felt it was all about him, and she was a vessel for his pleasure.

Having her concerns minimized so bluntly, Brenda lost momentum in bringing this sexual fantasy to life and she started seeing sex with her partner as more focused on his needs. When she stopped to think about it, he was dismissive of her feelings and needs in nonsexual aspects of their relationship, too, centering himself instead of holding space for mutuality in how they addressed their goals and obstacles together. It wasn't long after that Brenda realized she wasn't turned on anymore when he made advances. She brought up her concerns and he professed his apologies about dismissing her fears. But

> Brenda no longer felt safe bringing other people into their sex life.

In this case, it is clear that Brenda was struggling to feel safe enough with her partner, emotionally and sexually, and she had concerns about sexual safety if other partners were involved. Though she felt safe enough to stay in the relationship given her partner stopped minimizing and dismissing her needs, Brenda's desire for him had been on a steady low since this exchange.

Safe with Whom?

To be turned on, you must first feel safe enough with yourself, with partners or others, and in the world. These paradigms of safety are often intertwined in surprising ways, and it can be equally important to define what "safe enough" means to you in each area. Or you may find that your relative safety in any one of these contexts exceeds the others in terms of prioritization. Your comfort depends on your experiences in life and in the world as a result of your various identities.

How safe you feel with yourself when it comes to sex is often driven by temperament, previous experiences, expectation of resilience, and how much trust you have in yourself, and the resources and support you have at your disposal if something were to happen. When it comes to sex, how we feel about ourselves can set the stage for how well we protect our own well-being. You cannot predict or prevent another person from hurting or mistreating you. And there can be ways in which you may not be caring for yourself, which can decrease the level of attuned prioritization you have with yourself, often leading to disconnection from one's mind, body, and sexuality.

Women are often given the message that their needs, wants, and limits are second to those around them and they may have been given positive reinforcement for abandoning themselves and catering to others first. This can foster a relationship with yourself in which you deprioritize your needs, wants, and limits. To reestablish that relationship, it can help to develop a practice of self-reflection and mindful connection with your body and emotions—key ingredients to setting more sustainable boundaries.

Make no mistake, feeling a lack of safety with yourself is the goal of any oppressive system, because the more connected you are to your physical body, mind, and self, the more you can appropriately self-advocate and fight against its goal of keeping some people less powerful and sovereign, and in service of others. Doubting yourself and deferring to the authority of others (men) gives them more authority and power over you, your body, and your sexuality. In chapter 3, I discussed how trusting yourself was an essential part of healing from trauma, especially sexual trauma. Keeping women in a state of self-doubt and disconnection is a prime way to ensure that they are easier to manipulate and gaslight, and more likely to collapse when faced with the threat of not being safe. To begin to trust yourself, and to heal and advocate with confidence and agency for your sexual needs, the prioritization your own needs, limits, and boundaries is key. This means having an active dialogue with your body and emotions, and honoring the communication points that arise about what does and doesn't feel safe enough for you.

Practicing Safety with Yourself

How do you develop practices of safety with yourself? It sounds simple, but taking little actions regularly can build a feedback loop between your body and mind that you've got your own back and paying attention to yourself. Interoception (see chapter 5) is the name of this game, as it keeps you more connected to the cues of your body, so you can home in on how you feel and what you need, what you want or explicitly don't want in any given situation. Here is a list of exercises for you to try.

- Start with building mindfulness practices that draw your awareness to your body. Mindfulness exercises are a key instrument in developing a strong mind and body connection.

- Educate yourself on sexual health, anatomy, safer sex practices, and STI screenings, so you can decide what safe enough means to you in this context.

- Practice actively regulating your emotions. Learn different grounding techniques to help you keep your emotions in proportion to the moment. Emotions are of enormous value to your decision-making process, so the goal is not to minimize them, but to let them be informative without becoming overwhelming.

- Get enough rest. Rest gives our internal systems the ability to do what they do best and allows us the chance to be open and receptive—mostly to ourselves.

- Develop healthy approaches to communication and conflict resolution, which strengthen your ability to stay present and connected and facilitate assertiveness.

- Practice centering yourself. This doesn't mean ignoring the needs or limitations of others. It means checking in with yourself first, to be clear with yourself about your experience in a given moment or situation, so you can adequately respond, negotiate, or leave when a situation is no longer a good fit for you. Check back in with yourself after an exchange to see how you feel as a result. Checking in with yourself regularly is the best way to center your own experience.

- Seek support. While it may be tempting to think you can practice self-safety on your own due to the emphasis placed on individualism in Western cultures, knowing when you need help and seeking it out within your community and with professionals is essential in establishing safety with yourself.

Securing safety with others rests on your ability to cultivate safety for yourself. Being able to properly negotiate and advocate with others depends on you first having a fortified understanding of yourself and a willingness to trust that you can be OK walking away from a dynamic that does not align with your needs. You may or may not find that your attempts to get on the same page are always met with flexibility and openness from a partner.

Safety with Others

Establishing safety with a partner shouldn't have to be a rigorous and exhaustive process, but it can be, often because of power dynamics, earlier life experiences, and stressors in our everyday lives. Knowing how you define safety, or safe enough, gives you and a partner a good start to see where you are aligned in constructing a mutually safe-enough dynamic and where you might need to get some clarity to create alignment. Notice I said *create* alignment and not *find* alignment? No two (or more) people are going to be 100 percent aligned on everything. So, it's not a passive process of stumbling into a dynamic of safety. Safety is created through mutual understanding, curiosity, openness, and negotiation that respects the boundaries and needs of every party involved. If that's not the energy you're bringing (and seeing in return) already, you might pause and reevaluate.

People in therapy often ask how they can spot someone who may not be committed to developing mutual safety in sexual or romantic relationships. Here are a few tells, though this is not an exhaustive list.

- If someone disregards the need for informed and ongoing consent.

- If someone ignores, dismisses, or placates, and then violates your agreements or boundaries, sexually or nonsexually. In fact, most grooming behavior begins with nonsexual violations, to test whether or not someone will self-advocate or let the behavior slide.

- Any pressuring, guilting, manipulation, or coercion for sex. You don't owe anyone sex, for any reason. If you can't say no at any time for any reason, then your yes is invalid and there is no consent.

- If someone cannot or will not communicate openly about their desires, concerns, or boundaries, or about yours. It may not be malicious if someone does not know what they want or like, or what their boundaries are, but being able to name that is key to establishing safety instead of dismissing or stonewalling a conversation about it.

- Lack of transparency and agreement about safer sexual health practices and STI status. People have different levels of comfort around STIs and the risk of transmission, and that can be OK, depending on whether you are able to agree on what you both need to feel safe enough before embarking on sexual activity. But if someone refuses to share their STI status, get tested, or use contraception, or shames you for bringing it up as a request prior to having sex, or refuses to engage in safer sex practices that are important for you, the lack of compatibility is likely to reduce your sense of safety with them.

- Avoiding conflict is a big red flag, signaling that someone might not have the ability to work through hard things. At first it may seem like bliss to be part of a dynamic that seems so easy, but avoiding conflict doesn't mean there is none; it means there is no trust that you'll be able to successfully navigate the conflict.

This is a common adaptation for people who have not had safe strategies for handling conflict modeled for them, or who had to learn to fawn or appease others to stay safe in previous relationships. But it can lead to disrupted authenticity and a dynamic of placating and then erupting in passive-aggressive or aggressive rage.

- Neglecting or dismissing one's or a partner's needs or emotional well-being. Neglect is a quiet form of abuse and can be easy to overlook as it often comes without a big blowup or heavy confrontation. It may feel like being dropped in the middle of a bid for connection or it may be a partner failing to follow through on something they've agreed to do. Over time, it erodes trust and fosters an imbalance of power in the relationship.

- Chronically avoiding accountability or getting defensive when you bring something up is a warning sign that someone lacks the emotional regulation skills to handle feedback and make adjustments to their behavior that support the relationship or situation. It also shifts blame back to the aggrieved person and can be a strategy that abusive people employ to direct blame, maintaining a position of power while ironically playing the victim themselves. Does this person live in an echo chamber or do they have people in their life who challenge them and hold them accountable other than you?

- Failing to acknowledge, respect, or celebrate elements of individuality, diversity of identities, and experiences between partners. This is evidence of an enmeshed or rigidly egocentric mindset that can make it difficult for a person to have empathy for the plight of others.

- Hindering your personal and emotional growth or refusing to do their own work. It's important to assess your own goals and trajectory of growth and healing in life in both sexual and nonsexual areas. You and a partner may not evolve in the same way, at the same pace, or in the same direction, and that can be frustrating, but is not necessarily an indication that they are not a safe enough person for you. However, if they refuse to self-educate, reflect, or grow, or try to stifle your efforts to lean into growth or change, they may not have your best interests in mind or may be trying to control you for fear that your growth may signal the end of the relationship. Which, to be fair, it might. And that is a decision *you* may have to make—continue on your own path of growth and exploration, running the risk that your paths will diverge, or stay in a relationship with this person and feel truncated in your own self-development.

Building safety is not achieved in a vacuum and there are many external variables to take into account, including your community and the world at large. If you imagine your immediate community and the greater context of the national and global society, how safe do you feel in general? What about when it comes to sex? Many of us are subject to inadequate legal protections surrounding sexual violence or harassment, limited access to reproductive healthcare and sex education, discriminatory policies based on gender, sexuality, or relationship status, or stigma around exercising personal autonomy when it comes to sexual desire. Limited access to mental health services or support or to adequately trained professionals can leave people feeling vulnerable and limited in their self-advocacy. Further, being part of a community that is resistant to advocacy for sexual and relationship rights can make it dangerous for people to get legal support. Facing stigma or shame for discussing sex and relationships can leave people feeling isolated and hopeless. Being subject to rape culture or to a culture that does not prioritize consent practices can decrease a felt sense of safety or agency, and this contributes to the risk of sexual violence.

Am I Safe?

Each sexual experience is different and your needs for safety may change. You are dynamic and so are your needs for safety based on the experiences you've had in life and with a sexual partner. What may feel safe enough for you today may be different tomorrow. Or in five minutes. Safety is subjective and you get to define what it means to you.

Pleasure and desire come from a place of safety or calculated risk. There is an inherent vulnerability in pleasure and desire. If you are too closed off or protected, you might be successful in blocking out the majority of risk, but by blocking risk you might also be guarding against pleasure. It's not for me or anyone else to dictate your safety needs, only you, on your time frame.

Pleasure Points

- Feeling safe is integral to sexual desire and pleasure. Even people who incorporate risk or fear into their erotic life calculate a cost-benefit analysis to ensure the pleasure outweighs the fear.

- Safety in sex and relationships is better conceptualized as a continuum rather than a binary experience. Acknowledging the fluctuating nature of safety and risk are crucial for a nuanced and layered understanding of your own safety needs.

- The human brain has a tendency to perceive more threat, sometimes creating a negative perception bias, which can sometimes cause people to rush to judgment and miss out on opportunities for pleasure and sexual growth.

- Safety is subjective, and determining your sense of safety is a practice of staying connected to your somatic cues, thoughts, feelings, and behavior, to help guide a curious, empowered, and discerning sense of self-advocacy.

Pleasure Reflections

- What are some personal experiences that have left you feeling less safe, and how did you recognize those feelings in your body, emotions, thoughts, or behavior?

- Reflect on a situation where you had to negotiate desires and boundaries. How did you navigate it and how were your efforts received? How did that contribute to a sense of safety, or not?

- In what ways do you establish safety with yourself, in both sexual and nonsexual aspects of life? How does your relationship with yourself impact your overall safeguarding and well-being?

- Consider the red flags mentioned for identifying someone who may not have mutual sexual safety in mind. Have you encountered any of these behaviors with past or current partners? How did you (or would you like to) respond?

Chapter 8

Do I Have to Say Yes?

Two of the most insidious thieves of sexual desire are sexual entitlement and sexual coercion. And they are prevalent. Homing in on this point, Farida D., a prolific feminist author, opined, "Patriarchy denies women the right to be sexual; to experience sexual pleasure and to express their sexual desires—but at the same time expects women to be readily sexually available for men. This is not a paradox. It is exactly how things are supposed to be in a patriarchy. Women are not taught to *have* sex but to *give* sex to men."[1]

Sexual entitlement is rampant, and nearly everyone has participated in, witnessed, or experienced it. Research indicates that roughly 16 percent of women and 9.6 percent of men have experienced sexual coercion in their lifetime,[2] and these data are likely an underrepresentation of reality, given the lack of education about coercion and underreporting. Unsurprisingly, research shows that sexual entitlement has an inverse relationship with desire.[3] In other words, the more sexual entitlement one partner exhibits, the less desire the other partner is likely to have. In my time working with perpetrators of sexual coercion, I've noticed three defined response styles, which I've labeled "the defensive deniers," "the befuddled disbelievers," and "the entitled admitters."

This array of predictable responses exists because perpetrators of sexual violence often gaslight and minimize their behaviors in the hopes of managing your impression of them and clouding their accountability or consequences to maintain a path to reoffend. Shame prevents defensive deniers from envisioning themselves as a person who would engage in sexual violence. And they tend to refuse to see sexual coercion as violence, since they didn't use force. Befuddled disbelievers claim that they didn't know what they were doing was coercion. They thought their partner consented and didn't piece together the manipulation or force they used to coerce a yes. When they "get it" they claim to be horrified. And the third group of perpetrators, entitled admitters, generally don't believe their partner should have the right to say no, whether it be because they bought dinner, participated in household tasks, or see sex as part of the duties of being in a relationship. They generally see interactions as transactional and believe sex was a right being "withheld" from them. They often believe they were being abused, because they weren't getting what was "rightfully theirs," so their action is erroneously justified as righting a perceived wrong.

Author and survivor Natalie LaJune frequently discusses the effects of sexual coercion, and categorizes the perpetrators of coercive behavior as "soft" or "hard," differentiating between perpetrators who "don't realize they're doing it," and those who "do it without apology."*

---

*   Natalie LaJune is an author and survivor who founded alwaysmending.com, where she frequently writes about the effects of sexual coercion. Her quotes are shared with permission, via personal exchange.

Sexual entitlement is pervasive in patriarchal societies, given that patriarchy was created to control female sexuality in service of male power, social standing, and patrilineal passing down of wealth.[4] Galvanized by religious interests, sexual entitlement became enshrined as a declared right of men. That is not to say that only men engage in sexual coercion—that's certainly not the case—but this is how sexual entitlement became so prevalent and has led to rape culture, sexual double standards, incel communities, and outrageous (and yet still underreported) instances of sexual violence. Often rooted in gender and race-related power dynamics and imbalances, sexual entitlement and coercion are often used as a tool to reinforce dominance and a hierarchy of power, control, and authority, whether the behavior is committed intentionally or not.

Sexual entitlement and coercion are in direct opposition to consent, and any coercive behavior undermines any "yes" that is given. In order for consent to be valid, it must be freely given and mutual, and each party has to believe that there will be no negative consequences to saying no. When there is sexual coercion, entitlement and manipulation overtake any mutuality and center only one partner's desires and boundaries while disregarding those of the other.

What Is Sexual Coercion?

Coercion is a step beyond entitlement, but entitlement is always a part of the mix when coercion is present. Coercion is to use manipulation, pressure, or force to obtain sexual compliance. Notice I didn't say consent. It's not just physical, though, and here is where many people get tripped up on what constitutes coercive behavior—perpetrators and victims alike. Emotional manipulation can include guilt-trips, threats, refusal to participate in household tasks or activities, sulking, passive-aggressive comments, negging (a compliment that also includes a backhanded insult), intimidation, pressuring other family members such as kids, punishment in nonsexual contexts, and restricting finances. This is not a complete list, but hits on the most commonly used tactics to compel a yes, however tepid or obligatory it may be. Victims may comply to avoid negative consequences, but not out of any authentic desire. Here are some examples of verbal and nonverbal ways perpetrators may attempt to coerce you into having sex.

- **They may be demanding.** "I've waited long enough. We are going to have sex tonight."

- **They may ignore your boundaries.** "Come on, I know you really want it. Just go with it."

- **They may gaslight you.** "I never force you to have sex. You're crazy!"

- **They may objectify you.** "You look so hot—I want a piece of that!"

- **They may evoke pity from you.** "If you really loved me, you'd want to have sex with me."

- **They may decide unilaterally.** "I know what you like. I don't need your consent."

- **They may make you prove yourself.** "If you really care about me, you'll prove it by taking care of my needs."

- **They may apply pressure and guilt.** "I do so much for you and this family, can't you do this for me? Physical touch is my love language."

- **They may compare you to others.** "Other people have a better sex life than us, let's fix that."

- **They may make threats.** "If you don't have sex with me, I'll get my needs met somewhere else."

- **They may disregard your nonverbal cues.** Persisting in their behavior despite your signs of disengagement or discomfort.

- **They may engage in unwanted touching.** Groping or touching your body, without your consent, and in a way that is sexually stimulating for them.

- **They may try to get you intoxicated.** Plying you with drinks until your barriers evaporate or you can't say no.

- **They may ignore your safe words or gestures (a word, phrase, or signal agreed upon in advance to convey a desire to stop sexual play).** Disregarding or "pretending" not to hear/ notice your desire to stop in disregard of your boundaries.

- **They may engage in stalking behavior.** Following you in person or online with the purpose of compelling you to have sex.

- **They may share intimate content of you without your knowledge or consent.** Distributing your photos or content, for their own sexual gratification, in lieu of having sex, or to non-consensually get off on your sexual material.

- **They may try to isolate you.** Keeping you alone and vulnerable or refusing to let you leave so you'll have no means of help or escape.

- **They may get you gifts.** Buying you nice things or things you've wanted with the explicit and manipulative purpose of a quid pro quo* return on their investment.

- **They may ignore your discomfort.** Being unresponsive to your concerns or feedback that you are not enjoying what is happening.

- **They may try to humiliate you.** Making sexual advances in front of others to pressure your compliance.

---

* Quid pro quo is Latin for "this for that" and describes a transactional situation common in sexual coercion, where the perpetrator offers to do something nice for someone in exchange for sex.

- **They may be persistent.** They may consistently ask for sex, despite your repeated refusals.
- **They may create a dependency.** Creating a context where they are needed or relied on, and therefore have leverage to negotiate sex.

CASE STUDY

Content note: This case study includes descriptions of sexual coercion/assault.

Zoe was put on bedrest for the last three months of her pregnancy due to complications of her age and other health concerns. Her doctor specifically told her not to do anything that elevated her heart rate, including even mild exercise or walking more than from the bathroom to the bed. She felt defeated, as this was her first pregnancy and she had been looking forward to exercising all the way through—it was her favorite form of stress relief. Zoe's husband said he understood and told her he would help her by taking on more chores at home and bringing her dinner when he was back from work. Otherwise, she was left to work from her bed, and could get up briefly to get herself water or snacks. She was terrified to even do that much, as the doctor was specific that her heart rate could not be elevated.

Zoe's husband was great for the first week or so, but then he started asking about when they could have sex again. Zoe was appalled he was even asking, as if sex should be a priority for either of them right now, given the precautions the doctor specified. Zoe's husband retreated, but stopped bringing her dinner every night for the next week, claiming he "forgot." She was furious and accused him of pouting and not bringing her dinner intentionally. Her husband was incensed and told her that if she couldn't find a way to be sexual with him over the next few months, their relationship was going to suffer. What was he supposed to do, watch porn or find someone else to have sex with until the baby came?

Shocked and heartbroken, Zoe told her husband to do what he needed to do. So he climbed on top of her, penetrated her, and left the room after his orgasm. She couldn't sleep all night, shocked by the horror of what he had done, worrying about whether her heart rate had been too elevated given her anxiety, and then filled with more anxiety about whether her anger and worry might also hurt the baby. This happened every two or three days until the baby was born, and luckily the baby and Zoe were healthy. Zoe's husband persisted after she gave birth, and repeatedly claimed the six-week waiting period was nonsense and they were safe to have sex. At first, Zoe refused. But her husband came home one night and told her about his coworker whose wife had sex two weeks after giving birth and that she was "fine."

Zoe felt like a hole to be plugged and not seen at all for what she had just been through, or how her body was still trying to recover. Every night she refused to have sex, he refused to help with the baby and spent the evening hours watching porn, loudly, from the other room. Zoe had never seen this side of him and every ounce of desire she once felt for him disappeared. Even after the six-week healing period, Zoe felt no interest in having sex of any kind. He grabbed her hand one day and placed it on his penis, guiding her through manual stimulation. Six months later, she still had no interest in being sexual with him, and told him to go have an affair if he needed sex so badly. And he did.

I wish Zoe's story was anomalous, but it is a story therapists hear over and over. Zoe's husband believes he is entitled to sex and believes she should provide it to him. His petulant "forgetting" of her dinner and threats to go outside the marriage for sex if she does not comply are a clear example of an entitled admitter. He disregarded the medical recommendations assuring both a safe pregnancy and postpartum healing, putting Zoe and their baby at risk, so he could have a few moments of pleasure for himself when she was too weak and inhibited to take alternative steps to ensure her safety. He victimized her in one of the most vulnerable times of her life. One year later, she wanted to leave him, but still felt too weak to do it all on her own. She continued to report a lack of desire for her husband, as he had proven to be an unsafe person for her over and over again. She was repulsed by his touch.

Regardless of the motivation of the perpetrator, the effects on the victim (and the victim's future sexual desire) can be serious. It is common for survivors to experience symptoms of post-traumatic distress similar to those who have experienced sexual assault, since sexual coercion is a form of sexual assault in which one's consent is not feely given. During or after a coerced event, the body releases stress hormones (such as adrenaline and cortisol), which flood the system to prepare the body to respond to the threat, otherwise known as the activation of the hypothalamus-pituitary-adrenal

(HPA) axis. This stress on the body can result in muscle tension, pain, and reduced blood flow to the digestive system, which can leave you feeling nauseated, in urgent need of a bowel movement, or with an upset stomach.

The fight, flight, freeze, or fawn responses are all are expected ways one might respond to sexual coercion. There is no hierarchy of correct responses to threat, so please do not judge yourself for how you may have responded or reacted. The freeze and fawn responses are common responses to sexual coercion, and for good reason. Some coercive partners may escalate aggression or violence to overpower a partner's attempt to fight or escape the encounter.

The freeze response is an instinctive way to protect yourself from a perceived or real threat. The nervous system activates tonic immobility, which is essentially a playing-dead response. Trust and safety are key goals in secure functioning relationships, and in romantic or sexual activities. Coercion makes safety and trust near impossible, and a freeze response is a physiological reaction, not a conscious decision, to the overwhelming fear, stress, or danger present. The freeze response generally consists of a disconnect or feeling of detachment between mind and body, and may involve depersonalization (feeling distant), derealization (feeling as though one's surroundings are not real), or dissociation as the mind unconsciously attempts to minimize harm by refraining from engaging in any behaviors that may get a perpetrator's attention, like fighting back or trying to get away. (See chapter 5 for more about dissociation, depersonalization, and derealization.)

Similarly, the fawn response is about evading further risk and going along with what is being demanded so as to minimize the potential for further harm. This is an adaptive strategy in the moment, when it does not feel safe to assert or reinforce one's boundaries.

The subject of the coercion instinctively, and mostly unconsciously, acts in a way that appeases or pleases the perpetrator. This can look like being compliant with what is asked or demanded of you, or even actively anticipating and meeting the stated or perceived needs of the person displaying sexually entitled attitudes or behaviors. This can evolve into an ongoing pattern of people pleasing and prioritizing someone else's needs over your own, even when your limits are not aligned with their desires.

Some people who have responded with a freeze or fawn response feel shame or guilt, or even experience a sense of self-betrayal. This internal conflict is amplified if their body exhibits any signs of sexual arousal or orgasms. Arousal non-concordance (ANC) is common during sexual abuse and assault, and is a discrepancy between how a person's genitals react to stimulation and whether or not they actually *want* the sexual stimulation. When genitals are stimulated, they don't always have connection to conscious thought and they respond whether the touch was wanted or not. This is why some people report experiencing lubrication, an erection, pleasurable sensations, and even an orgasm despite being vehemently opposed to what is happening; it is stimulation without consent. **Genital arousal does not mean the sexual stimulation was wanted or consented.** Please read that last sentence again.

Another example of arousal non-concordance is when someone's mind says yes for sex, but their body is not responding with the typical signs of sexual arousal, as is the case for some sexual dysfunctions.

Many people who have experienced arousal non-concordance feel especially betrayed by their bodies as there is often an erroneous belief that one should be able to control the body's reaction. It's natural to want to believe that we have control in a situation where we are overpowered. Genital arousal when consent has not been given, or there is no conscious desire, can be a survival mechanism, elicited unconsciously to prevent or minimize injury from penetration or additional harm. It is essential to know that genital arousal in coercive situations does not equal desire. Perpetrators may weaponize your body's survival response and goad you with comments that suggest you really do want to be sexual. This is simply not the case, and is a myth perpetrated by rape culture. When determining your comfort, willingness, or consent, subjective arousal—meaning your active desire and interest in sex in that moment—should be prioritized over any physiological reaction in your body. Not the other way around. Cognitive dissonance is common after experiencing arousal non-concordance. Trust yourself. If you did not want to be sexual and your body responded anyway, that does not mean you "secretly" wanted the sex that was being coerced. Remember to have empathy for yourself and the part of you that is wise and working extra hard to keep you safe in moments of sexual discomfort, distress, or duress.

Antithesis to Desire

If this chapter resonates with you, there are many reasons you may have lost desire. When you encounter sexual entitlement and coercion, its impact lands in the body, calcifying as an emotional defense against desire. It is difficult to feel trust, connection, or safety with a person who considers their own sexual needs above your humanity. Constant pressure from a partner to be sexual can chip away at autonomous desire and feed a sense of obligation, resulting in a somatic shut down (hypoarousal). Internalizing a negative view of your freeze or fawn response or arousal non-concordance can make you lose trust in your own body and instincts.

Losing trust or confidence in the partner who maintains an entitled attitude or has engaged in coercive behavior is also likely, although it can feel as though you are in the wrong for questioning their intentions. Why would you trust someone who doesn't respect your agency? How a partner responds when you bring up your discomfort is key to understanding whether they have humility, empathy, or care for you. Maybe it happened just once, as they severely misread the situation. Sure, maybe. But if it happens again, and in some cases again and again and again, it is healthy to question whether you can really trust this person and your safety around them. If your desire has become extinct after entitled or coercive experiences, your body is screaming NO by redirecting energy to survival instead of desire.

It is common for coerced partners to avoid intimacy altogether, associating feelings of helplessness, powerlessness, betrayal, disgust, or fear with sexual encounters. If someone stays with a partner who has been coercive in the past, but is now reformed and no longer exhibiting that behavior, it can still take a long time for the coerced person to feel truly safe and embodied around their partner in both nonsexual and sexual situations. Even if you choose to move on and partner with someone new, it can take time until you feel safe enough to be sexual.

However frustrating it may be to you or your partner, it is better for you and your desire to refrain from obligatory sex, or from sex because of pity, guilt, or any worry they may leave. Engaging in sex when you are not truly interested in being sexual communicates an overriding of your body's cues, which can extend the process of healing and reconnecting with desire authentically.

The emotional numbing and detachment that allowed you to get through the coercive encounter can continue for a while, making it difficult to connect with pleasure, joy, or even to be clear about your own emotions or physical sensations. If the power imbalances remain unresolved in your partnership, a cycle of chronic disempowerment can render it difficult for you to stop numbing out emotionally, as that may be protective for you in the moment. Healthy communication and boundaries are necessary for desire and mutual, pleasurable sexual experiences. It's difficult to communicate with a partner who is emotionally immature, coercive, or otherwise abusive when it comes to sex or your agency. While numbing your emotions is an adaptive strategy in the moment, over time it can suppress desire immensely.

What Can I Do to Stop Coercion?

You are not responsible for someone else's behavior, and you can't control how someone else chooses to behave. What you can control is how you react and proceed once someone has shown themselves to be coercive, but only when you feel safe enough to take some action. This timeframe is yours to determine. No one knows your predicament better than you, so trust your instincts. The following few steps can help you make sense of your options and decide what path is best for you.

First, establish your emotional, physical, and sexual boundaries (you may want to explore these first with yourself and then with your partner; see chapter 15 for more about this). Once you are clear, be firm and assertive in your communication about what you are and are not OK with. Clearly express your lack of consent, assuming you feel safe enough to do so, using unambiguous language. If necessary, or preferred, you may want to remove yourself from the immediate situation and give yourself and your partner some distance to process. If you have safety concerns, it may be best to develop a safety plan with a professional or someone else you trust, to ensure you have support and help ready to call upon. You might consider developing a code word with a friend or supportive ally, so they know when you are in distress and your plan of action is needed. This may sound easy, but these steps can feel overwhelming, scary, or impossible. Take your time. Self-advocacy is taking action when you feel ready to do so, not according to someone else's agenda.

Pleasure Points

- Sexual entitlement and coercion are prevalent throughout society. Perpetrators are often defensive, minimizing, or further entitled when confronted.

- A result of patriarchal conditioning, sexual entitlement is a key component of rape culture, sexual double standards, and instances of sexual coercion and violence.

- The principles of valid consent and sexual coercion are in direct opposition, as coercion involves manipulation, pressure, guilt, or force to extract compliance.

- Victims may respond to coercion with a fight, flight, freeze, or fawn response. All are healthy adaptations to a threatening event and can lead to post-traumatic distress symptoms.

- Coercion and sexual entitlement can result in somatic shut down (hypoarousal) and emotional numbing, which can reduce desire and lead to avoidance of sexual experiences.

Pleasure Reflections

- Have you observed any signs of sexual coercion in any of your sexual or romantic relationships?

- How do you communicate your sexual boundaries to someone and appraise their response?

- If you have experienced coercion, how has it affected your feelings of trust, safety, or desire with that partner, or other partners?

Chapter 9

Do I Feel Desired or Objectified?

A few years ago, I hosted a panel discussion for women and femme folks to discuss various aspects of their experiences with sex. One of the questions I posed to the panel was, "How do you know when you feel desired or objectified?" The impetus for this question is from a wave of social media content I had witnessed in the preceding year that focused on women discussing the first time they experienced catcalling or unwanted male attention. Most of the women who had spoken of their experience recalled being prepubescent or pubescent when they noticed men's comments or sexually charged behavior. Some were as young as three or four. As mentioned in chapter 3, early experiences of sexual abuse or violation can have effects lasting into adulthood. Many people do not think of being objectified at a young age as a form of abuse, but when objectification happens, either to children or adults, it can be confusing, disturbing, and uncomfortable.

In response to my question, there was a mixture of blank looks, somber stares, and a couple of women who were eager to jump in. Interestingly, many women in the audience conflated these experiences, and interpreted the objectification they experienced as being desired. Can both things be true? I suppose. But I'd argue that the feeling is different. Desire often feels like an invitation. If you put up a boundary, desire respects and redirects. Objectification often feels like an intrusion or a violation of sorts. Like you're being used and not seen. For many people, especially women and people AFAB, the experience of being objectified or desired by others is how they are introduced to their own sexuality. Like many of the women on the panel, and many women in the world, differentiating between one's own desire and the experience of being desired can be a confusing journey. Add the feeling of objectification and it can lead to a decrease in desire.[1]

Chronic sexualization and objectification position women to experience their own desire through and secondary to their partner's desire. This is especially reinforced in heterosexual relationships, because women's pleasure is frequently deprioritized (hence the orgasm gap). For centuries, women have been discouraged from knowing and centering their own desire and the effect is that they often experience it *when* they are desired. It is not a biological or inevitable truth that women experience desire only when they are desired, but one conditioned into women through shame, sexual entitlement, double standards, and the desexualization of women who become mothers, change in physical appearance, or dare to age. Dr. Wednesday Martin speaks to a different reality, and notes that female sexual desire is thought to be far more expansive and fluid than male sexuality, but due to patriarchal restrictions, it is often reduced to a one-dimensional understanding and purpose: providing pleasure.[2] If that is not your template for arousal, well, you might feel pretty unaroused when providing that pleasure.

In this minimized and reductionist view, women's desire is activated when someone else desires them. That is the only time when being sexual is acceptable. But what if you stand in your own sexual agency and declare what you find hot on your own terms? Some people might raise their eyebrows and discourage you from declaring it. This ensures that women's sexuality remains under the control of others and thwarts their sexual autonomy. And what if being desired is what turns you on? That's completely OK. What turns us on is a mix of biological and environmental factors, and it's not always politically correct.

Desire is a complicated process that feels simple by the time we're conscious of it. Think back to chapter 2, about identity. Desire is often connected to identity and can either affirm a sense of self or offer access to a taboo that's opposite to our presented self. Look at those who are drawn to dominatrices: many are well-accomplished, successful men, with a lot of responsibility in life. Desire in their play as subs gives them access to a tabooed experience of self—the person they cannot afford to be, a person with little to no responsibility, who gets bossed around (and sometimes humiliated), and doesn't have to think too hard about holding it together for anyone. It's a release to be outside the position of power you are expected to demonstrate in real life.

We can glean that the same is true for many women. Responsible for disproportionate amounts of emotional labor and the sexual pleasure of others (in many cases, men), countless women feel as if they can finally let go and surrender to pleasure when the focus is completely on them. Being desired is one way that women are told they are worthy, but their beauty is often seen as a symbol of social status for their partner, making them valuable (in a patriarchal society). To be desired in this way is then to become commodified and it can be difficult to discern, especially in heterosexual relationships, when a woman is desired for who she is versus what she does for a man.

People of all genders are capable of internalizing an objectified view of their worth. In a social system that is structured hierarchically, those arbitrary variables of worth are also attached to power. Women of color and those in other marginalized groups or bodies experience this fetishization and objectification at rates even higher than those in bodies deemed most socially acceptable—the thin, white, less-curvy body. There is a long history of how these -isms (such as racism, sexism, ableism) have corrupted humans' relationship with power, access, and desire, and it is beyond the scope of this book.[3] However, the effects are widespread.

These hard truths bring up strong defenses for some people, but it's important to acknowledge them. We may not be able to eliminate the objectification that is all around us, but we can look at how it impacts desire. No two people have had the exact same experience, as our identities and social experiences vary. It's up to you to decide if and how much objectification has shaped your relationship with sexuality, and whether it could be a part of why you may find sex less accessible.

CASE STUDY

Jordyn was excited for her best friend to meet her new partner. They'd been dating for almost a year, but her best friend had been away at school and just returned. The two women planned a dinner date with their partners and a few other friends. Jordyn's partner liked to drink and so did her best friend, so she thought they'd at least be drinking buddies. Jordyn's best friend was ferociously protective of her and had a critical eye when it came to men. Jordyn worried that if they didn't get along it would make life challenging.

During dinner, Jordyn's boyfriend made a toast to her best friend, and everything was going well, so far. But as the dinner went on and the drinks started flowing, Jordyn's boyfriend became more and more affectionate. His affection was endearing at first, but Jordyn could sense his desire was building. He got very horny after a few drinks and was really sexually disinhibited. Their sex life has been incredible up to that point. But toward the end of the meal, Jordyn stood up to toast the table, and her boyfriend reached up behind her, in front of everyone, grabbed her breasts and said "MINE!" before slamming another drink.

Jordyn's best friend rolled her eyes and told Jordyn, "No." Jordyn was confused; he was just expressing his desire and didn't mean anything by it. She loved that he was so affectionate and didn't hold back showing how much he wanted her. But Jordyn's BFF could immediately see what she would learn over time: that her partner had a tendency to objectify her, and his desire was not for her as a whole human, but for what she represented to him. Jordyn eventually felt this as a devaluation of her humanity, not just sexually, and the relationship ended. But about six months before she ended the relationship, she stopped feeling any desire for him. He was livid and became incensed when she pointed out that it wasn't a turn-on when he would make objectifying gestures. He would often balk at her, and reply, "Please *objectify* me! I'd love to feel *objectified*, even once!"

Their exchange showcases how insidious and unconscious objectification can truly be, and how it is so often embedded in the way sexual desire is confounded with gender and power. For many men, to desire is to objectify. Even for men who do not display sexual boundary violations, the language of rape culture and objectification seeps into their psyche in their early years, evading conscious perception. So, too, can it infiltrate how women and nonbinary people experience desire and being desired with cunning stealth.

When I write about objectification online, it's common for men to chime in that they would "love to be objectified," therefore women should appreciate their overtures. However, if I'm in a teaching mood, I will reply and ask them if they want to feel objectified or desired. Those men who enter the conversation in good faith will often respond that they want to feel desired. To which I offer, of course they do! Everyone wants to be desired! But most people, unless it's part of their kink, don't want to be objectified. Because being desired factors in your humanity. It respects your individuality, your autonomy, your unique experience, and choices. Objectification does not. Objectification strips the desired object of their humanity and renders them inanimate.

To be clear, everyone is capable of objectification. It is a necessary part of early human development: Before infants develop the cognitive sophistication to understand their caregivers are whole, separate humans, they make sense of them as objects that fulfill their needs. We develop the ability to move past objectification to seeing people as whole in our early childhood years. Well, some of us do. Othering is a form of adult objectification. It's easier to be cruel and to subjugate others when you see them as less human, or not even human at all.

The Difference Between Desire and Objectification

When desire is reduced to a predefined set of characteristics it is, at its core, objectification. This is why desire can feel confusing. You may not always feel objectified when in fact that is what is happening. And you may feel objectified or sexualized, even if that isn't someone's exact motive. Intent and impact are different! Objectification occurs when a person is treated like less than a human, like an object. They are seen as devoid of their individuality, their autonomy, and their agency, and their desirability hinges on how well they satisfy external expectations, rather than their actual desires. In other words, they are desired if they fit the mold of what they are expected to be—if they are compliant with the expectations of their dehumanization. If someone has a rigid expectation that their partner has long hair, because only long hair is appealing to them, should their partner cut their hair (and exercises agency, autonomy, and bodily sovereignty), they may be unconsciously perceived as too human, as someone with a voice and needs and not solely for use. Objectification is about power, and when it is the way some groups of people have been taught and rewarded for treating other groups of people, it can become difficult to disentangle from desire.

Feminist scholars who have studied objectification point to a framework that highlights ten inherent capabilities of human beings, as outlined by Martha Nussbaum, which, when restricted, reduce their agency, autonomy, and overall well-being. It's these capabilities that make us human and different from literal objects.

10 Capabilities of Humanness[4]	10 Features of Objectification[5]
Life: the capability to live a full and healthy life, encompassing the need for nutrition, shelter, and medical care	**Instrumentality:** treating another person as a tool or object for one's purposes rather than as a subject with agency; reducing an individual as a means to an end
Bodily Health: the capability to have good health and physical integrity, including control over one's own reproductive and sexual functions	**Denial of Autonomy:** disregarding a person's autonomy and agency, treating them as lacking self-determination or the ability to make choices
Bodily Integrity: the capability to control one's body and to be free from assault or coercion, including the right to make choices regarding one's sexuality	**Inertness:** perceiving someone as passive, lacking in agency, and incapable of independent action or initiative
Senses, Imagination, and Thought: the capability to use one's sense, imagination, and thought in a manner that is informed and fulfilling, free from oppressive restrictions	**Fungibility:** viewing individuals as interchangeable or substitutable, ignoring their unique qualities or individuality
Emotions: the capability to have emotional attachments and experiences, fostering connections and relationships with others	**Violability:** considering a person as violable, that is, treating them as an object without boundaries or inviolable rights, thereby subjecting them to mistreatment or harm (being violated)
Practical Reasoning: the capability to engage in critical thinking, make informed decisions, and participate in political and moral decision-making	**Ownership:** seeing a person as owned or controlled by another, implying a lack of independence or self-possession
Affiliation: the capability to live with others, forming meaningful relationships, and participating in a social community	**Denial of Subjectivity:** treating a person as though they have no subjectivity, and do not have unique feelings or experiences that matter or need to be considered
Play: the capability to enjoy recreational activities and leisure, contributing to a balanced and fulfilling life	**Reduction to Body:** focusing on a person's physical attributes to the exclusion of the other qualities, such as intelligence, emotions, or personality
Control over One's Environment: the capability to participate in the community and to have control over one's political and material environment	**Reduction to Appearance:** treating someone based on the qualitative assessment of their appearance and how they appeal to one's senses
Other Species: the capability to engage with the world and other species, recognizing the interconnectedness of life	**Silencing:** seeing a person as if they are silent or lack the capacity to communicate verbally or nonverbally

In reality, the evidence of objectification can be subtle. People who objectify others aren't always doing it consciously and they are likely to deny that objectification is the basis of their actions because (1) most people don't understand the subtleties of objectification, and (2) they don't want to think of themselves as actively engaging in a dehumanizing position. And yet, women experience a tremendous amount of objectification, whether just existing or in romantic and sexual contexts. Consider these examples by comparing them to the Features of Objectification to see if any apply to you.

- **Overemphasis on your looks:** Compliments are focused on your appearance, instead of your other characteristics, personality traits, or interests. (Reduction to Appearance)

- **Ignoring your personal boundaries:** Your boundaries or discomfort are disregarded to fulfill their needs or desires. (Instrumentality, Violability, Denial of Subjectivity, Ownership)

- **Limited interest in your inner experience:** You rarely engage in conversations about your thoughts, feelings, ideas, opinions, or values. (Denial of Subjectivity, Silencing, Denial of Autonomy)

- **Exclusively sexual conversations or lack of emotional connection:** Conversations and interactions are consistently driven to a sexual topic or purpose, at the expense of learning about, or participating in, emotional intimacy or other aspects of your life or inner experience. (Instrumentality, Silencing, Denial of Subjectivity)

- **Using you for validation:** They seek validation from others, primarily through showcasing your appearance (and sometimes other achievements). (Instrumentality, Inertness, Reduction to Appearance/Body)

- **Ignoring your interests or refusal to engage in shared activities:** No curiosity about your passions, hobbies, interests, or goals is expressed, or you participate in activities only they like to do, while disregarding your interests. (Denial of Subjectivity, Denial of Autonomy)

- **Disregarding your feelings, gaslighting, or dismissiveness:** Your feelings, achievements, thoughts, or contributions are ignored, minimized, or dismissed, or the context or situation is manipulated in such a way to make you doubt your inner truth. (Denial of Subjectivity, Inertness, Denial of Autonomy)

- **Maintaining a transactional approach:** They view their interactions with you as a series of exchanges and transactions, with a focus on what they get out of it. (Instrumentality)

- **Ignoring consent or failure to respect consent:** Engaging in any activity (especially sexual) without your clear and ongoing consent, or pressuring, manipulating, coercing, or guilting you to engage with them beyond your boundaries. (Instrumentality, Denial of Autonomy, Inertness, Violability, Ownership, Denial of Subjectivity, Reduction to Body)

- **Expecting your availability:** They assume you are always available for and to center their needs, without regard or reciprocity for your priorities or needs. (Denial of Autonomy, Inertness, Ownership, Denial of Subjectivity)

- **Treating you like a possession or isolating you:** They act as if you are a thing they own or have control over, or they try to keep you to themselves, away from friends, family, or your community. (Denial of Autonomy, Instrumentality, Silencing, Inertness, Ownership, Denial of Subjectivity)

- **Reducing you to a set of stereotypes:** They refuse to see your individuality, and instead see you through the lens of stereotypes attributed to your characteristics (i.e., race, ethnicity, gender, age, etc.). (Fungibility, Inertness, Denial of Subjectivity)

- **Conditional praise or positive reinforcement:** They show affection, attention, or positive reinforcement only if you conform to their expectations of you. (Instrumentality, Ownership)

This is not an exhaustive list of examples, and you may see additional links to the various features of objectification beyond those listed. How many have you experienced in relationships or interactions with sexual partners where your desire for them or for sex in general has waned?

Being objectified can take a gnarly toll on your mental health and detract from your capacity to fully lean into feeling and expressing desire. The experience of sexual, emotional, or physical objectification can leave you feeling disconnected from your own inner wellspring of sexual agency, authenticity, and pleasure. After all, if you are being treated as someone whose inner experience doesn't matter, as a tool for someone else's pleasure or productivity, like something that can be violated or destroyed, or like something only as important as its physical appearance is pleasing, there is a high likelihood of your experiencing dissociation, difficulty establishing self-protective boundaries, anxiety, and pressure to perform to the role you've been assigned. Talk about a libido killer.

Do Women Objectify Themselves?

This is a complicated question. Women can internalize the objectification they have experienced, and act according to the expectations they believe are to be fulfilled. Adopting what is sometimes referred to as "the male gaze," women can become spectators of themselves, watching to ensure they are conforming and performing to the expectations and desires put upon them. In that sense, yes, women can self-objectify. Self-objectification might look or feel like any of the following.

- Seeking a partner's approval of your appearance before deciding if *you* like how you look
- Chronically prioritizing your partner's desires and needs over your own
- Engaging in performative behavior at the expense of your authenticity and conforming to an expected role for approval or validation, like moaning loudly to feign pleasure
- Disconnecting from your own pleasure or quieting your own desires
- Comparing your appearance or sexual prowess to others' and believing you are only worthy if you meet the expectation set by the comparison
- Overemphasizing sexual behaviors to conform to others' expectations of you
- Having a difficult time with self-advocacy.

If you recognize any of these tendencies, do not be harsh with yourself. You can decide if you want to challenge yourself to move away from self-objectification or not. Now that you can better recognize objectification, you might begin to track if and how you experience it from others, or within yourself, as well as the impact it has on you, if any.

Is It OK If I Like to Be Objectified?

I might ask you, after reading this chapter, is objectification really what you mean? Or do you mean desired? Do you mean free to surrender to pleasure and have someone else take the reins? Many kinky people love to play with dehumanization and objectification, and part of why it feels so good to them is because their humanity is factored into their consent—and *it is play*. Their humanity is respected in how a kinky scene (the structured play session between consenting adults) is negotiated. In it, their boundaries are respected, their experience and desires solicited and honored, and each play activity is designed to be of mutual benefit. To play with these themes can be erotically charged, for sure! But the key word here is *play*. It is erotic because it's a fantasy, not a reality. To be objectified in reality often comes with real existential, financial, emotional, or physical consequences. It can be soul-destroying unless it is a transactional agreement entered into by consenting adults. But even in those cases, the toll of chronic objectification often looms large and can be in conflict with true desire.

To be sexualized or desexualized are two sides of the same coin, because both reveal a role someone has been put in, a silencing of their needs, and a stripping away of their humanity and individuality. Many women find themselves feeling invisible sexually. As they age, their bodies change, or they have children (and now fall into a different role in service to others). People can be sexual at every age, and it is through their dehumanization that this reality is denied. While they may not be sexually objectified, the *emotional* objectification continues, in the form of inequities in emotional and domestic labor. There is still dehumanization afoot in emotional objectification, because often the person being objectified is seen only as an instrument for another's emotional regulation or for meeting their everyday needs.

With this deeper understanding of the many facets of objectification, in what ways have you been objectified by a partner or by another human?

Pleasure Points

- In this patriarchal society, women experience a tremendous amount of objectification, which can have serious implications on their desire and arousal.

- Desire encompasses a person's humanity and acknowledges their internal experience, autonomy, and uniqueness, whereas objectification reduces a person to their physical appearance or a specific function and denies their individuality.

- The experience of objectification can impact people of all genders and sexual orientations, race and ethnicity, and physical size, shape, and ability, though women of color and other marginalized identities frequently experience more and in more extreme forms.

- Objectification can limit women's sexual autonomy and agency, reducing their experience of desire and pleasure to a performance for the approval of others.

Pleasure Reflections

- Reflect on your experiences in society, in relationships, and sexual interactions. Consider how you have felt valued for your holistic self, individuality, and desires, or how you may have been objectified. Can you detect a difference between the two?

- Consider how it feels to be genuinely connected to your own sexual desires and interests, separate from the desires of a partner.

- In what ways might you be participating in the objectification of others, or yourself?

Chapter 10

Are We Compatible?

One of the biggest grifts about love and sex is that when you find "the one" everything will align. Your "person" will be the perfect piece to make you whole and vice versa. However, partnerships become a terribly disappointing reality when your idea of an ideal union is that you have to be in perfect alignment, each of your quirks harmoniously complimenting one of your partner's oddities. Perhaps nowhere does this romanticized idea of relationships hit harder than when it comes to sex. With sex education so lacking, coupled with an expectation that the quality, frequency, and kind of sex you have as partners means something about the strength of your partnership, many partners find themselves shocked and afraid when there is a mismatch in their level of desire. But there is no "normal" when it comes to sexual frequency, interests, or desire, despite some aspects being more common than others. There is tremendous diversity across the human experience in physical ability, appearance, taste in food, musical preferences, and so on, and that diversity extends to sexuality, too.

We Want Sex at Different Times

Of course you do! You're different humans, with different biological, social, emotional experiences and demands. When polled, 80 percent of couples reported wanting sex at different times,[1] proving how commonplace it is to be on a different erotic clock than your partner. There may also be biological factors at play that make you horny at different times. People AMAB frequently report enjoying sex in the morning due to higher testosterone levels at that time, whereas people AFAB conversely report more desire in the evenings. This is likely due to feeling more relaxed. However, as people age, many gravitate toward sex earlier in the day, as their schedules tend to lean toward earlier mornings and bedtimes. Variances in desire are not always due to differences in biological sex (and hormones), but can be related to different energy levels and circadian rhythms (internal sleep–wake cycles that oscillate every twenty-four hours).[2] Natural circadian rhythms influence when a person has their peak moments of energy and alertness, and when they start to get fatigued. Are you a morning person and is your partner a night owl? Vice versa? Neither is good or bad, but it can make syncing up for sex a more consciously timed experience. What scripts might you be carrying around about to trigger the right time for sex?

Conflicting work schedules, personal, social, or familial responsibilities, and diverse time management routines can make it tough for partners to align their schedules with enough time to be emotionally or sexually intimate. How many times have you and your partner plopped down after dinner and sat in silence as you decompressed from the day's stress? One of you may recharge enough for sex after a short stint of your most recent TV binge, while the other may need more rest or even a full night's sleep before having the energy for sex. Sleep preferences can make for inhospitable sexual ambience and can influence each partner's desire and sexual willingness. What is the state of your bedroom? Your bed? Is this a space where you both feel erotic? If not, what would you change?

CASE STUDY

Vera and Megan had been together for close to five years. Vera was frustrated that they rarely had sex spontaneously, unless they were on vacation. Megan was also annoyed, but said they should schedule sex, so they could be better prepared, energized, and in sync. Vera hated this idea and said it felt "forced and obligatory" to schedule sex.

The idea that scheduled sex is off-putting is a common retort when sex therapists make the suggestion that partners carve out time intentionally for the possibility of intimacy. Another ingrained belief, thanks to cultural and media narratives, is that desire is always spontaneous and felt to the same degree at the same time. And if it's *not* spontaneous, then it *must* mean something about the quality of your connection. But most of the time it doesn't mean anything more than that you have different internal clocks, and a little coordination can help you protect some time for the possibility of sex. You don't have to make it a mandatory exercise. Instead, create time for touch, set the ambience, or play a game together. Be consciously present and active in your intentions, giving yourselves time and space to build to sexual intimacy if you're both feeling it.

How Much Is Enough?

The right amount of sex to be having is the amount of sex all partners are interested in having. For one couple, once a week may feel ideal. For another set of partners, four or five sexual encounters each week is the best amount. At the end of 2023, my clinical practice, Modern Intimacy, conducted a poll of our online community, asking about many aspects of people's sex lives over the year. While 23.7 percent reported not having a consistent partner, 17.8 percent reported partnered sex once a week, 22.4 percent reported partnered sex two to three times weekly, 3.9 percent noted partnered sex was a daily activity, and 32.2 percent endorsed having partnered sex less than once each week.[3]

Because desire and pleasure are so subjective, wanting sex at the same frequency can also cause concern between partners. Desire discrepancy is a leading cause of frustration for partners, alongside money and parenting conflicts.[4] The higher-desire partner can feel like a nuisance, ashamed that they seemingly always want sex more than their partner, or can be sensitive to being rejected. They may resent being the primary person to initiate or feel concerned that their partner is saying yes only out of obligation. The lower-desire partner may feel shame or guilt for not aligning with their partner's needs, or they may feel pressure to say yes to avoid hurting their partner's feelings. Unresolved for long periods of time, both the lower-desire partner and the higher-desire partner can begin to feel inadequate, undesirable, unloved, or burdensome. It is common to avoid the conversation altogether when partners are trying to avoid disappointment, creating gaps in a once strong emotional connection, and resulting in less overall sex.

Many other factors influence desire, including general health, side effects of medication, changes in hormones, as well as ideas about one's identity. Even thoughts about how much more or less sex you think you *should* be having can be a factor. Many partners worry that variety, novelty, and relationship satisfaction are at risk when there is a discrepancy in desire. But remember that there are no normal or designated limits when it comes to desire. Female sexual desire is often misconstrued as being lower as a result of biological differences, or it's seen as lower compared to assessments of male sexuality (see chapter 1). In fact, people born in female bodies have comparable levels of desire to those born in male bodies, after confounding variables, like stress, are accounted for.[5]

If you or your partner suddenly experienced a shift in desire, a good place to start is by investigating any contributing factors. For example, have your schedules changed? Is one of you getting less sleep? How can you support each other to rebalance?

CASE STUDY

Tatum was deeply in love with their partner, Noa. Their relationship blossomed after a work trip brought them together from opposite sides of the country. They dated long distance, and after about a year, Tatum decided to move from NYC to LA so they could live together. During their first year together, their sex life was rewarding and easy. They experienced a lot of spontaneous desire for one another. But about six months after moving in together, Noa noticed that Tatum seemed less frequently in the mood. They planned sex, went on dates, and Noa worked hard to infuse romance into their day-to-day life. Tatum was appreciative of Noa's efforts, but just didn't feel desire as frequently. During couples therapy, they were invited to say the first number that came to mind when they both imagined their ideal frequency for sex. Noa quickly stated, "Four or five times a week." Tatum was shocked and started to cry, before saying to Noa, "You must be so disappointed

in me." Noa comforted Tatum, assuring them it was not
the case. As they explored, Noa learned that Tatum barely
participated in solo sex more than once every other week.
When they were dating long distance, they had no metric
to assess their libidos in real time since they often met for
long weekends where there was little to no stress and lots
of excitement and novelty— a recipe for lust! Now that they
lived together, there was less dopamine driving their desire
and Tatum's baseline was clear. Tatum expected when they
moved in together they'd both settle into a cadence that
felt less intense, because while they loved the sex they had,
sex was the last thing on their mind after working ten-hour
days.

Tatum and Noa took an honest look at how they
managed the demands of their jobs, their finances,
domestic tasks, social time with friends and family, time
together, and solo time. They also looked at their sleep
routines and body clocks. Tatum was an early riser but
got tired as the day went on and was early to bed. Noa
was just the opposite. Though they both worked from
home, Noa's workday started around 10:00 AM and was
over by 4:00 PM, and that's when their day really started
to get going. The couple realized that Noa had a lot of
time for hobbies and exercise and felt more desire in the
evening. Tatum had very little time for any self-care, given
the demands of their work. Typically working East Coast
hours on the West Coast, their workday started at 6:00
AM and was typically over around 5:00 PM. Then Tatum
usually made dinner and cleaned up. Tatum loved to cook,
and didn't see this as a burden, but when they looked at
how they could preserve energy for sex, both partners
agreed that Noa would take over dinners three times per

week and have it ready by 6:00 PM, so they could spend time unwinding. Because Noa woke up later than Tatum, Noa volunteered to do the dishes the next morning, too. Rebalancing their stress and to-do lists gave them both designated time to connect. They didn't push the agenda of sex, but within a few weeks, Noa started to notice they had more bandwidth for sex after the pair started taking walks after dinner.

Many partners fall into the trap of assuming the desire discrepancy is one person's problem to solve. However, like Noa and Tatum, when they work collaboratively and get creative in their approach to the problem, acting like players on the same team instead of two players on opposite sides, they can find a way back to desire. Sometimes the collaboration is, in fact, the magic. Working together with curiosity, empathy, and a judgment-free approach will help you catalog the reality of your lives before you determine if the desire discrepancy you are experiencing is finite. If supporting each other differently gives you space to curate more time for sexual intimacy, how could you shift your day-to-day activities? Sometimes partners will push back against the idea that they have to do more chores or take on more responsibilities to *earn* more sex. To which it warrants questioning, is sex a transaction? Are you currently stuck in resentment that prohibits you from moving out of a tit-for-tat exchange? Do you think your partner wants to do those chores or have those responsibilities either? Probably not. What would it mean to your partner to know that you were on the same side of the problem, showing up for each other to get to a common goal? Perhaps that is a more erotic (and sustainable) mindset.

We Don't Have the Same Turn-Ons

It's not surprising that mismatched sexual interests between partners can lead to a misalignment of preferences and desires, leaving one or both partners dissatisfied. In order to find a middle ground, partners must be able to communicate without judgment or fear of rejection. Having different turn-ons can be a net positive in a relationship, especially if the partners involved have a relatively flexible arousal template, meaning they can be aroused by a wider variety of stimuli. You can share and participate in each other's preferences and enjoy a wide array of sexual variety.

But that isn't always the case if one or both partners has a fixed arousal template, feels unsafe, or cannot get into what the other likes. They may feel inadequate to please their partner, and also stuck because they don't want to participate in a sexual act that they can't get their head around. Feeling pressure to avoid disappointing or hurting their partner, they may compromise and go against their own limits, only to have their discomfort confirmed. While it can be awesome to push yourself along a growth edge, doing something sexually that you are not comfortable with is likely to create more distance than resolution for you and your partner. Alternately, if one partner's fantasies or preferences are consistently being overlooked, minimized, or dismissed, it can make them feel unseen, not valued, or that their pleasure is deprioritized.

CASE STUDY

Selah's partner loved to be restrained during sex. Selah didn't understand this at all, as she was "pretty vanilla" and thought putting her partner in restraints was for domineering women, not for her. Selah's partner felt disappointed because he really trusted Selah and hadn't felt so open to exploring his desires in a long time. Selah was adamant that this was something she could not participate in, but she didn't know why other than it "didn't feel right" to her.

Upon further inquiry, Selah was able to identify that during sex, she was most turned on when they were engaged in mutual play. Putting her partner in restraints felt like a one-sided activity where she didn't get any pleasure but had all the responsibility. In therapy, she discovered that as an eldest daughter, she didn't want to have to be in charge of someone else's experience, since growing up, she was often tasked with having to manage everyone around her. Being in this role sapped her erotic energy and desire and left her feeling resentful of her partner.

Selah's partner understood but felt dismayed. He wondered how they might be able to both be satisfied and realized the appeal of being restrained was that it was the only time he felt free from the obligation of taking care of others. Selah got teary; she knew her partner's family relied on him a lot, too. She never looked at restraints in that way before and wondered if she also might like it. He asked her what might make her feel like it was a mutual exchange. Selah thought about it, and replied that it would feel more mutual if he was pleasuring her while restrained. Her partner lit up with excitement. He brainstormed ways he could pleasure her while restrained, taking the emotional labor off of her, and found a face mask with a built-in dildo. He knew Selah loved being penetrated, so he surprised her and bought it. He also suggested that only his feet or hands be restrained at a time, so he could move enough to kiss and pleasure her in other ways. They agreed to give it a try, and to their surprise, felt carefree and also mutually engaged.

If your fantasies don't line up with your partner's, consider the deeper underlying desire. Once you understand if the discrepancies and preferences are about obtaining a specific kind of sensation, an experience of power or surrender, or something else, it can be easier to discuss fresh ideas on how to align you both.

We Are at an Impasse

Sometimes partners just can't get on the same page sexually. It happens, and if that's where you are, know that it doesn't necessarily mean anything about who you are as people or how much you care about each other. Sometimes a period of enforced celibacy, in which abstinence from sex is not a desired outcome, is just where you are at—sometimes temporarily and sometimes permanently.

If you're really at an impasse and finding a middle ground for your sex life is impossible, there are a few things left to consider. You can't change each other, so stop trying. Really think about whether the relationship is one that will work for you in the long run, and if this is as good as it gets. It's a tough reality to consider, but a necessary step for your own sexual health. How important is sex to you in this relationship? What might it look like for you not to have exactly the sex life you'd imagined or hoped for? Is that a bargain you're willing to make, to protect the rest of the relationship? If not, then you might want to consider uncoupling to give yourself and your partner a chance to create a relationship with someone else where more of your needs are met sexually. If so, here begins the process of grieving and redefining.

In the alternate situation, it's OK to grieve the sex you'll never have. When I once posted this on social media, I was floored by the number of people with whom it resonated. You may love your partner, but feel sexually unfulfilled. Grief is an important step to generate options for having a better sex life. Sometimes we get stuck in the unprocessed grief of not getting what was expected or wanted, and it limits our solutions for other forms of pleasure or vitality.

There are also other options for staying with a partner when you have mismatched desire. Might you be satisfied exploring areas of sexual mismatch on your own, through solo sex? Perhaps you might consider opening your relationship, so you or your partner can experience what you can't get from each other. Perhaps porn is an outlet that could suffice? What safeguards would you and your partner need to have in place to feel comfortable with an expanded concept of sexual pleasure?

In having this conversation with your partner, it's essential that neither of you agree to anything that feels like self-abandonment. So often, a fear of losing the relationship leads to a choice that abandons your own wants, needs, and limits. Shortly thereafter, the sex that you agreed to starts to feel obligatory, unsafe, or becomes fodder for resentment and disconnection. When you're making changes with your partner or on your own, it's best to start super slow and to reevaluate frequently to ensure you're making an intentional decision that reflects an embodied connection.

Pleasure Points

- The idea of perfect sexual alignment is a myth. It is natural for there to be some diversity in what partners like or how frequently they want sex.

- Biological, emotional, social, and relational factors all play a role in determining desire. Personal schedules and routines, along with stress levels and circadian rhythms, can influence readiness for sex.

- Divergent sexual interests that remain unaddressed can lead to sexual dissatisfaction as well as emotional hurt and relational disconnect.

Pleasure Reflections

- How have cultural, religious, or media influences shaped your expectations of sexual compatibility? In what ways might some diversity in sexual interests benefit you and your partner?

- Reflect on your and your partner's libidos. What external factors, if any, are influencing any discrepancy? If there were changes that could be made to remedy barriers to desire, what might they be?

- How important is sex to you in a partnership? What about it feels important to you? What do you believe it means for you or about you, if it is not as important to your partner?

Chapter 11

Am I a Partner or a Parent?

Finally! You've found your person and you're building the partnership you've always imagined. Or something close to that. Partnership has always been the dream—someone you truly get and who gets you, and who you work with to build a life and strong relationship. Somewhere along the line though, it stopped feeling like a partnership. Instead, you've started feeling more and more responsible for everything: getting groceries, planning dates, starting hard conversations, teaching your partner how to show up for you, making sure the kids have their homework ready, and generating the energy for sex. You're exhausted and your relationship feels one-sided. No wonder you feel short on desire!

Do you feel like a partner in your relationship, or do you feel like a parent?

When I ask this question to clients in session, their response is generally a mix of validation, horror, anger, and despair. For some, this question puts words to a feeling they haven't been able to name and it's the first time they're seeing their relationship dynamic through a different lens. For others, this question validates what they have been saying to their partners, over and over and over again, and despite multiple attempts to bring it up, they have seen little movement to reshape the dynamic at home, leaving them frustrated, disconnected, disinterested in sex, and isolated.

What did you notice in your body when you read the title question for this section? Did you see it in the table of contents and then skip ahead to read this chapter first? What is this phenomenon all about? Why is it so pervasive? And what does it have to do with desire?

Well, a lot. Especially in heterosexual relationships.

The Unequal Labor to Low Desire Pipeline

When one partner is consistently doing more work than another, it can lead to a whole host of relational challenges, especially decreased desire. Feelings of resentment, fatigue, or a lack of trust in one's partner can be some of the nonsexual impacts of labor inequities, and it can also result in waning sexual interest. The two most common ways this can show up in relationships is through an unequal division of emotional labor and an unequal approach to domestic labor.

I FEEL LIKE MY PARTNER'S PARENT/THERAPIST

Emotional labor in relationships refers to the effort and energy invested in managing and nurturing emotional well-being—both your own and your partner's. It involves activities such as active listening, providing emotional support, empathizing, and addressing conflicts sensitively. Emotional labor is essential in healthy relationships. It fosters emotional intimacy and connection, creates a safe space for vulnerability and open communication, and strengthens the bond between partners. This enables them to better understand each other's needs, fears, and desires. Emotional labor helps in conflict resolution. It allows couples to navigate disagreements constructively, leading to healthier resolutions and preventing unresolved issues from festering.

Inequities in emotional labor often arise due to societal norms, gender roles, or personal expectations, and can emerge in relationships when one partner consistently shoulders a disproportionate share of this responsibility. This can lead to feelings of resentment, burnout, and ultimately, relationship dissatisfaction. Recognizing these imbalances and addressing them through open and empathetic communication is vital to maintaining a healthy and equitable relationship. Emotional labor should be a shared responsibility, fostering mutual growth, understanding, and satisfaction within the partnership.

Two especially insidious versions of gendered emotional labor are sexual emotional labor—"the other third shift"[1]—and hermeneutic labor.[2] Hermeneutic labor is a specific kind of emotional labor that entails knowing and expressing your own feelings, desires or wants, goals, intentions and motivations with skill and accuracy, being able to discern and interpret them in others (especially a partner), and anticipate and generate ideas and solutions for interpersonal conflict or tension. Sexual emotional labor refers to the emotional work women perform during sexual experiences to protect their partner's ego, sense of self, or confidence, including faking orgasms, tolerating sex that is uncomfortable or painful, defining sexual satisfaction on their partner's pleasure or experience of satisfaction (even if their pleasure was not equitable), or accepting sex they determined to be bad as acceptable because their partner expressed satisfaction. This form of emotional labor is called "the other third shift," to reflect an additional late shift of unpaid labor that can exist in romantic and sexual relationships. The first shift refers to paid work outside the home. The second shift denotes the unpaid domestic and caretaking labor that occurs when someone gets home from their paid job.

Not sure how emotional labor plays out nonsexually? Here is a list of twenty examples of other ways inequities in emotional labor might be present in your relationship.

Initiating Communication: one partner consistently initiates conversations about feelings, while the other rarely does

Remembering Dates: one partner remembers important dates, like anniversaries and birthdays, while the other often forgets

Apologizing First: one partner always apologizes first after an argument, regardless of who is at fault

Supporting Through Tough Times: one partner is there for emotional support during difficult periods, but the other is absent or dismissive

Planning Dates: one partner is responsible for planning all the dates and outings

Managing Household Emotions: one partner is primarily responsible for managing the emotional climate in the household

Resolving Conflicts: one partner takes on the burden of resolving conflicts and making amends

Listening vs. Talking: one partner dominates conversations, while the other listens more often than they speak

Parenting Emotional Support: one partner takes on the majority of emotional support for the children

Comfort During Stress: one partner provides emotional comfort during times of stress, but the other doesn't reciprocate

Remembering Details: one partner is expected to remember all the important details about the relationship and the family, such as which child likes which brand of cereal

Expressing Vulnerability: one partner feels comfortable expressing vulnerability, but the other hides their emotions

Taking Care of Friends and Family: one partner takes on the emotional labor of maintaining relationships with friends and extended family

Conflict Avoidance: one partner avoids conflict at all costs, while the other must navigate and manage it

Expressing Gratitude: one partner rarely expresses gratitude for emotional support, leaving the other feeling unappreciated

Mental Load: one partner carries the mental load of managing schedules, appointments, and responsibilities, causing emotional exhaustion

Household Chores: one partner is responsible for organizing and delegating household chores

Navigating Social Events: one partner is expected to handle the emotional labor of socializing, such as making plans with friends and attending events

Decision-Making: one partner is always the one making major decisions in the relationship

Managing Insecurities: one partner is expected to constantly reassure the other about their love and commitment

I DO EVERYTHING AROUND THE HOUSE

Domestic labor encompasses the various tasks and responsibilities involved in maintaining a household, including cooking, cleaning, grocery shopping, childcare, and more. It is a fundamental component of any partnership, as it ensures the practical and logistical functioning of a shared living space and promotes harmony, balance, and overall well-being. Without it, your home doesn't run! Sharing domestic labor demonstrates mutual respect and cooperation between partners. It signifies a commitment to working together to create a comfortable and organized living environment, reducing stress and fostering a sense of unity. Moreover, equitable distribution of domestic labor is necessary to prevent resentment and conflict within a relationship. When one partner shoulders a disproportionate burden, it can lead to feelings of inequality and frustration, potentially eroding the relationship's foundation.

Inequities in domestic labor often arise as a result of unspoken agreements rooted in societal expectations, traditional gender roles, or communication breakdowns. There may have been an explicit agreement that is no longer working, as life or the amount of domestic labor required to keep your home moving has changed. And that is to be expected! People, relationships, and families are dynamic entities, so renegotiating domestic labor is normal, especially as more and more homes rely on both partners' incomes to stay afloat.

It's essential for couples to openly discuss and negotiate these responsibilities, considering each partner's strengths, preferences, and availability. Establishing a fair division of labor along these lines not only contributes to a harmonious home but also reinforces a sense of partnership and shared responsibility, enhancing the overall health and longevity of the relationship. Nevertheless, many partners run into roadblocks when they bring up the conversation. Dismissiveness, invalidation, or placating thwart progress in the discussion, and usually leave partners feeling unseen, unappreciated, exhausted, and without any hope for change.

Whether there are inequities in emotional or domestic labor, the underlying effect is the same: inequities in power. Ironically, the partner not doing their fair share will often voice feeling disempowered and as if their partner is "nagging" them. These partners give away their power and play the victim role, claiming their partner "does things better" or "knows what to do" or should "just tell [them] what to do and [they'll] do it." The term for this is "weaponized incompetence," and it can be infuriating to witness over and over again. Weaponized incompetence is a manipulation in which a person pretends to be less capable or incapable at completing a task so they can avoid doing it. The result is that it forces another person, in this case their partner, to have to take over the mental load of managing the task and completing it. It is insidious, and if you've ever felt like it would just be easier for you to do something yourself instead of having to re-do a task after your partner attempts it, you may have been the victim of their aim to shirk responsibilities in the future. Common examples can include the following.

- A partner insisting they don't know how to load the dishwasher the way you like, so they don't want to "do it the wrong way," or intentionally doing it "wrong" to prove they will do it below your standards

- A partner pretending they can't comfort a crying or fussy child, or dress the child appropriately, and passing the child off to you to take care of those tasks, or intentionally doing these things poorly, resulting in a distressed child who they know will activate you to take over

- A partner claiming they are bad at planning dates, leaving you in charge of always planning activities or ensuring you have fun things to do together

Weaponized incompetence is not sexy.

How Does This Affect Desire?

Your partner is certainly wondering how this affects your desire for sex because they've likely chipped in here and there, and have begrudgingly taken care of the thing you asked them to do (after many harried requests), and they don't understand why their valiant effort didn't translate into an immediate romp in the bedroom. Yes, that is sarcasm you're reading.

Emotional and domestic labor are notoriously undervalued. In fact, studies have found that the economic worth of the unpaid domestic labor of women totals trillions of dollars annually, if it were compensated appropriately.[3] In other words, if you're doing a disproportionate amount of emotional or domestic labor, you're working for free. There are laws aimed at preventing labor exploitation in the workforce, but in many relationships, women are expected to do unpaid labor. Much of these expectations come from gender essentialism, which erroneously attributes different skills to people because of gender, when in fact, people of all genders are capable of doing all kinds of work—including domestic and emotional work.

Even when this labor is approached with equity, it can have an impact on your body. It's a lot to handle sometimes! But especially when you feel you're doing too much, and more than your share,[4] it can have a significant impact on your allostatic load—the cumulative wear and tear on the body as a result of chronic stress.

When one partner in a relationship consistently bears the brunt of emotional and domestic labor, it can lead to chronic stress and burnout (see chapter 4).[5] This stress can stem from the constant juggling of responsibilities, feeling overwhelmed, and the emotional toll of unaddressed issues. A high allostatic load can lead to various physical health issues such as fatigue, insomnia, and chronic pain.[6] These ailments can be physically exhausting, making it difficult for you to find the energy and motivation for sexual activity. Feelings of sadness, hopelessness, or constant worry can consume your thoughts, leaving little room for sexual intimacy. Over time, chronic stress can elevate cortisol levels in the body, leading to long-term health problems, and can have a profound negative impact on sexual desire within a romantic relationship. Further, chronic stress can cause a hormone imbalance, reducing the production of sex hormones like testosterone, which are crucial for sexual desire.

Unequal distribution of emotional labor, such as always being the listener or emotional caregiver, can lead to mental health challenges such as anxiety and depression. Likewise, domestic labor imbalances can result in feelings of resentment and frustration, contributing to emotional distress. These mental health issues, when left unaddressed, can exacerbate allostatic load and can lead to a decrease in libido.

Another affected area is body image and self-esteem. High allostatic load can manifest as hypertension, obesity, or increased inflammation, all of which are risk factors for serious health conditions such as heart disease and diabetes. Weight gain, skin problems, or other physical changes related to stress can make you feel less confident about your body, affect one's sense of self-worth and desirability and, consequently, less interested in sexual activity. If you're not feeling good about your body, it's difficult to feel good (and gain pleasure) *in* your body.

Inequities in emotional and domestic labor can strain the relationship itself. In some cases, the partner who is doing most of the emotional labor may feel as though they are in a caregiving or parental role rather than a romantic one. This shift in roles can dampen desire, as it's not conducive to romantic or sexual attraction. Constant arguments, misunderstandings, and feelings of unfairness can lead to a breakdown in communication and emotional intimacy, causing a hostile environment that makes it difficult for partners to feel desire for one another.

When one partner consistently bears the burden of emotional labor, it can lead to feelings of disconnection. This lack of emotional intimacy can reduce the desire for physical intimacy, as emotional connection often serves as a foundation for sexual desire. The resulting resentment, a libido killer (as detailed in chapter 6), can create emotional barriers that hinder desire and make it difficult to engage intimately with the other person.

When one partner consistently avoids sharing their emotions or doesn't reciprocate emotional support, it can create a sense of emotional unsafety, hindering the development of trust and vulnerability which are vital for desire and intimacy. The partner doing more emotional labor may start to feel undervalued or unappreciated, and the partner doing less may feel like they cannot meet their partner's expectations.

Chronic relationship difficulties can become a unique form of stress, further contributing to an individual's allostatic load, which can further strain the emotional connection between partners. When people are overwhelmed with stress, they may become emotionally distant or preoccupied with their own concerns, moving into a mode of self-preservation. This emotional disconnect can result in a decrease in desire.

To mitigate the impact of these inequities on allostatic load, partners should engage in open and honest communication. Addressing these issues together, redistributing responsibilities, and seeking support through therapy can help create a more balanced and less stressful environment. This might look like reading the book *Fair Play*[7] together and revisiting how you conceptualize tasks and their completion. In the book, author Eve Rodsky highlights the benefit of couples working together by outlining three key components of creating equity when it comes to domestic labor. She notes that coming together to fully understand the "conception," "planning," and "execution" of each task can help you both identify how to get on the same page. Ultimately, an equitable distribution of emotional and domestic labor can not only improve the well-being of each partner but also promote a healthier, happier relationship. Reducing the allostatic load through addressing these inequities can contribute to a longer and more fulfilling life together.

Here are some questions you can start with to help tease out an unequal approach emotional and domestic labor.

- Who is primarily responsible for tasks in the day-to-day management of our home, such as cooking (which meals), laundry, grocery shopping, cleaning, yardwork, auto maintenance? How often do these things occur? How long do they take? What is involved?

- Who typically initiates and plans activities to support your couple/family life, including scheduling appointments, managing finances and budgeting, and coordinating social activities or family events? How often do these things occur? How long do they take to coordinate? What is involved?

- Who is generally responsible for tracking the emotional needs within your partnership or family, providing that attunement and emotional support, handling conflicts, and managing the overall emotional and relationship health of your unit? What is involved? How often is this task performed?

CASE STUDY

Grace came into my office, exhausted. She cried for most of the first session because it was the first time she had space to focus on herself in years. She couldn't even use the bathroom uninterrupted at home without one of her kids or her husband, Nick, barging in with a question or need. Grace tried locking the door to get a little space and privacy, but she quickly realized that when she wasn't available to her kids, they were left unsupervised, due to her husband's inattentiveness. He wasn't a "bad father," she'd say out loud, as if to convince me and herself simultaneously, he was just busy. He worked outside the home and was always checking work emails, managing his work commitments, or watching TV trying to decompress. She was a stay-at-home parent, and the default parent, so this was her job, right? She'd tell him she needed support, and he would say OK, but nine times out of ten, his support was only verbal and did not become action. She was fried and frustrated.

Recently, Nick started complaining that they weren't as sexually intimate as they used to be. Grace couldn't remember the last time they'd made love or the last time she even thought about sex. She wanted to be intimate with her partner, but when she thought about having sex with Nick, she felt either nothing, dread, or "icky." Exploring these feelings further, Grace noted that she often felt as though she had three children: her two daughters and her husband, like she was taking care of him as much as of the kids. She noted that Nick rarely planned any dates, and when she brought up date night, he often said, "Sure, what do you want to do?" leaving her to make the plans.

She begged Nick to make the plans as she had a lot on her plate as it was, but he would counter by saying he didn't know what she would be in the mood for at dinner, so she should pick because he was "easy to please." She reflected to me in session that she often didn't know what she wanted to eat because most of the time she was so busy with the kids that she didn't have time to stop and think about what *she* wanted. She wanted Nick to step in and take some of that mental load away by making a decision for them (and showing her he knew her as a separate person).

Grace also asked Nick to help run interference with his parents, as Nick's mother had a lot of opinions about how Grace and Nick should be raising their little ones, which did not align with their parenting approach. Grace's mother-in-law frequently criticized Grace, but not Nick, for the food and activities they planned for the kids, and she didn't respect Grace's requests to stop offering unsolicited advice. Nick brushed it off when Grace brought it up with him, and would say things like, "She's a mom, too, just let her feel important." Grace felt that she was on her own, and yet she was still confused about why she felt very little desire for her husband.

As Grace learned more about weaponized incompetence and how emotional and domestic labor tasks can become unequally managed, she began to feel rage. Weeks in therapy helped her to process her anger over feeling exploited, disappointed, and exhausted. She brought her anger to the surface and was able to set some different boundaries with her husband and mother-in-law, taking more time for herself. After a while, she realized her husband was not stepping up. Though she was disappointed yet again, this was the information she needed to make some big changes. After another year in therapy, she decided to file for divorce. Her husband was baffled, and claimed this "came out of nowhere," which solidified to Grace that she'd made the right decision. After all, his claim was yet another example of weaponized incompetence and she was done. After her divorce, she met someone new and felt revived in her desire when she observed that her new partner self-initiated difficult conversations, support around the house (and he didn't even live there), and planned about 50 percent of their dates and activities. This parity gave Grace the space she needed to see her herself as a partner, not just a parent, and that was really, really hot.

Grace's story is so common, especially in heterosexual relationships. While there are many wonderful partners out there, there are many who enter into marriage or a long-term relationship with the belief that they do not have to show up in a meaningful way—that their physical presence is enough. Secure functioning partnerships exist on several principles and one is shared power and authority.[8] A partner who does not participate equitably and collaboratively is exerting power and exploiting the other partner through their passivity. Being exploited is not sexy.

Recognizing What's Happening

Sometimes inequities in emotional and social labor are easy to spot. But other times, patriarchal conditioning renders women so intrinsically responsible for what happens in their home and relationship that they don't see the exploitation that their body feels. Here are fifteen thoughts that are common for women who are doing a disproportionate amount of emotional labor.

- "Am I being too demanding by expecting more emotional support from my partner?"
- "I feel like I'm carrying the weight of this relationship on my shoulders."
- "Why am I always the one to initiate conversations about our feelings?"
- "I wish my partner would notice when I need support without me having to ask."
- "Is it unreasonable to want my partner to be more emotionally present?"
- "I'm tired of always being the one to apologize and make amends after an argument."
- "Does my partner even realize how much emotional labor I'm doing?"
- "I'm starting to feel emotionally drained and neglected in this relationship."
- "Should I bring up this issue with my partner, or will it just lead to more conflict?"
- "I miss the days when we used to communicate and connect more deeply."
- "Am I sacrificing my own emotional well-being for the sake of this relationship?"
- "Is it time to have a serious conversation about the unequal distribution of emotional labor?"
- "I deserve a partner who is willing to put in the same effort I am."

- "I don't want to feel like a parent or therapist to my partner; I want a true partner in this relationship."
- "What steps can I take to address this issue and find a healthier balance in our emotional connection?"

Great, One More Thing I Have to Do

Addressing these disparities is essential to maintaining a healthy and satisfying intimate relationship. Open communication, a willingness to share emotional labor, and working together to create a more equitable partnership can help rekindle desire and intimacy. Addressing high allostatic load and its impact on sexual desire often involves both individual self-care and therapy and couples therapy. Learning stress-management techniques, such as creating and maintaining different boundaries, practicing grounding, breathing, or relaxation exercises, trying different communication strategies and emotional regulation techniques, and focusing on improving the overall quality of the relationship, can help reduce allostatic load and rekindle sexual desire within the context of a loving and supportive partnership. It can feel daunting to put in more effort when you're already depleted, especially if your partner has not been meeting your efforts equally or in a way that feels effective or restorative. Unfortunately, nothing changes if nothing changes. This does not mean you have to take on a disproportionate amount of labor in perpetuity, but it may mean finding a balance between rest and continued individual and collaborative effort.

HOW DO I GET MY PARTNER TO CHANGE?

You can't change your partner if they're not willing to. But for those partners who are willing, and perhaps need a little more insight or understanding, you are already on the path to change. Naming the problem, defining it, and addressing it together are the first steps. Many partners can see the bigger picture, and while they may not love the idea of doing more by rebalancing the scales of emotional and domestic labor, they see the merit in doing so for the health of the relationship. In order to rebalance, try sitting down together and generating a realistic list of the breadth and scope of labor tasks. So much labor is invisible. You might want to tell your partner that you need them to take over groceries, but that alone likely won't alleviate you of the mental load necessary to keep track of what groceries are needed, with what frequency, which brands are favored by the family, which stores have better prices, and so on. Mapping out the invisible labor and deciding together what constitutes a good enough completion of the task is key to ensuring good communication about what needs to change.

WHAT IF MY PARTNER ISN'T WILLING TO CHANGE?

A tragedy in a relationship is having a partner who can't or won't be influenced by your needs. Sometimes a partner's lack of concern is fueled by narcissistic traits, entitlement, or rigidity around roles. Lack of empathy, lack of perspective, and egocentrism can also inhibit a partner from taking their overfunctioning partner seriously enough to make changes. (When you have a parent/child dynamic with your partner, it can sometimes be referred to as an overfunctioning and underfunctioning dynamic, to illustrate that one partner is not doing their fair share, and the other partner compensates by doing more than their fair share to facilitate the relationship.) Some partners will say they care enough to make a change, and then do it poorly, or don't follow through at all, only to have a tantrum when they are called out—sending you right back into the parent role. If this is your reality, there are a few dynamics to consider. First, you may be experiencing a form of emotional abuse, a version of abuse that employs words, actions, or behaviors to manipulate, isolate, undermine, or exploit you. If it is safe to do so, consider working with a therapist to help establish different boundaries or develop an exit strategy.

Let the law of natural consequences take over. In other words, what happens if you stop overfunctioning? What can you let go of? Who cares if the clothes pile up a little more? Who would get dinner started if you didn't? Can you uncouple your identity from the imperfect tasks that go undone or half-assed? What reality about the relationship are you denying by overfunctioning? Are you and your partner really as good a fit as you hope? Or does your overfunctioning keep you distracted from a reality you may not be ready for—that your needs are not being met and this relationship may not be good for you any longer?

If you keep coming back to the thought, "But it's my role," know that it's not. And if you're so upside down with inequities, then the rules need to be reimagined. Reclaiming desire is about making room. You are responsible for creating that space, even if your partner doesn't help. If you change, the system changes.

Pleasure Points

- Inequities in emotional and domestic labor can lead to resentment, feelings of overwhelm, and fatigue, which can negatively impact desire.

- "Weaponized incompetence" is a term that refers to the manipulative behaviors someone employs by pretending to be bad at something or pretending not to know how to do something to get out of doing that activity. This behavior exacerbates a lack of equality in relationships and is exploitation.

- Emotional abuse can negatively impact a person's self-worth and well-being, and is often involved when a partner engages in weaponized incompetence.

- Sexual emotional labor is emotional labor exhibited in sexual situations to protect a partner's ego.

Pleasure Reflections

- How do you feel about the current distribution of emotional and domestic labor in your relationship?

- In what ways might you want to advocate for a more balanced distribution with your partner?

- How might your partner (or you) engage in weaponized incompetence to avoid getting out of both the labor and the accountability?

- What, if any, examples of emotional abuse might you be experiencing in your relationship? How might that be impacting your desire?

- What boundaries or limits can you set to protect your well-being, emotionally and physically, and to set the stage for a healthier and more equitable relationship?

Chapter 12

Are We Even Attracted to Each Other?

Relationships evolve over time and periodically benefit from reevaluation. Even therapists and sex therapists struggle with desire and sometimes with knowing exactly how their relationship is changing. It happened to me. After a few months of feeling no interest in sex with my partner and feeling no desire or attempts to initiate from him either, I asked him, "Are you even attracted to me anymore?" I wasn't sure how I felt, because physically, I found him very attractive, but I had no interest in being sexual with him or in sex at all. When we first connected, we both eagerly initiated sex. We reveled in how great our sex life was together—the most synergistic sexual pairing we'd each experienced. But when the lockdown started, we were suddenly living together, and he started initiating sex less and less. After reflecting, we can now identify the cause of his withdrawal as conflicts in our relationship that had sent him on his own growth journey, but this wasn't obvious at the time.

What was obvious was that I wasn't interested in being the only person to initiate sex. That didn't turn me on, and it was starting to feel like a disparity in sexual emotional labor. After I dropped my bombshell question, my partner immediately assured me he was attracted to me, but that he didn't feel sexy. We'd become a little too comfortable ordering in dinner and watching TV after work. Without our usual routines at the gym, both of our bodies changed. The change in lifestyle, energy, and the experience of living in bodies that felt different really affected how we both felt in our own skin. I didn't care about the changes to his body, but still felt no desire because of how *I* felt in mine. He felt the same, unable to access desire because of how he felt in his. I was also burned-out, having started a new business in 2020; had realized I was in peak perimenopause; and had been left without my typical pre-pandemic self-care activities like socializing with friends, traveling, going out for dinner, or heading to the gym or a yoga class.

But despite our efforts to understand our shifting (nonexistent) desire, nothing changed. Without an active sex life, we were beginning to feel a little too familial, like roommates. And I wondered if my attraction to him (and his to me) was changing because we were, in fact, too familiar? Surely, if we both still found each other attractive, we'd be motivated to do something about it, right? Like many partners who work from home simultaneously and are around each other 24-7, we were comfortable together—maybe overly comfortable. The way we related to each other had changed. In addition to working from home, sheltering in place limited the social lives that once provided us so much physical and emotional space. Although our physical attraction remained intact, I began to wonder if perhaps our emotional attraction had changed.

Long-term relationships go through predictable phases, though their intensity and timing ranges from couple to couple. Attachment styles, early life experiences, previous relationships, values, expectations, health, and current life stressors and joys all influence the trajectory of a relationship. A key piece of that trajectory is desire, which is also influenced by these variables over time because we're layered beings and desire does not exist in a vacuum.

Let's take a closer look at the stages of a long-term relationship.

THE LUST PHASE

First, the lust phase. Everything your partner does is fodder for a romp. They look at you a certain way or touch your leg during a movie—nothing much is required for you to be turned on. The lust stage is governed by novelty and lots of dopamine! Testosterone and estrogen are also elevated during this stage, as the primary evolutionary goal is to get partners together to increase the odds of mating.

In modern society, there are many reasons for people to get together beyond a goal of procreation, but lust plays a huge role in overcoming disgust. As I mentioned in chapter 2, disgust is an essential emotion for protection. It helps us stave off people or ideas that may be harmful. During sexual encounters, we are exposed to a lot of biological data from a partner, and that data can be compromising to our senses or health. Smells, sounds, textures, sights, tastes—our bodies are in such proximity! Lust helps overcome some of the variables that may trigger disgust if we were to encounter them with someone else—someone we are not attracted to. Our olfactory senses are on high alert during sex, and without the dopamine that results from lust, it is easy to be turned *off* and deterred from the smells of close contact. Not only is lust fun, it's functional!

The lust phase of a relationship can vary in duration, but generally wanes with less novelty and more familiarity in the relationship. During this time, the lust drive supersedes any of the other drives (romance or attachment) and it is difficult to really get a sense of long-term compatibility with a partner, given the near constant elevations of dopamine that saturates your brain, along with testosterone, estrogen, adrenaline, and serotonin.

THE ROMANCE/LIMERENCE/MERGING PHASE

Around the nine-month mark, new experiences with your partner are fewer and farther between, and the dopamine in your brain is less intense. The lust drive becomes less active, paving the way for the romance or limerence (an "infatuation" or intense longing for another person) drive to take the lead. During this second phase, the primary goal is merging your lives together, securing a connection. This stage can last anywhere from month nine up to two years of partnership. During this stage, there are often bigger steps taken to solidify a "we" from a "you and me." Partners begin to blend their lives, meet each other's close circles of friends and family, and may move in together, get engaged, get married, or get pregnant. Each of these milestones is significant and represents another shift away from two individuals to a unit, a system of humans in partnership. It isn't necessary to experience each of these milestones to give the system of partnership shape and form, but they are common and can represent novelty and signify commitment. In this stage of a relationship, novelty wanes, and with it so does dopamine.

THE ATTACHMENT PHASE

More commitment, more fusion, and less novelty can be amplifiers of safety, which is necessary to enter into the third phase driven by the attachment drive. In secure functioning partner systems, the attachment phase gives way to new levels of trust, safety, connection, and satisfaction. Starting around roughly the two-year mark in a long-term relationship, the attachment phase is your carrier for the duration of a partnership. This is when you signal to the world, to each other, and to your own nervous system that you now represent each other's primary attachment figures in life. As a result, a new community or family system is alive and well. Governed by oxytocin, vasopressin (which together aid in building trust and connection), and serotonin, partners in this phase feel the sweet calm of protection from mutual investment. Closeness and emotional intimacy rule the roost and partners often feel content in their commitment. However, closeness and safety often come at the expense of novelty—and without novelty (and novelty's good friend dopamine), attachment can feel, well, boring.

Of course, this isn't the case for everyone, and that sense of excitement or boredom can ebb and flow, but attachment and lust are inherently at odds. Before you panic, being in the attachment phase is not incompatible with lust or romantic desire. Attachment is just the more primary drive, and the default drive of long-term relationships, as our long-term partners become attachment figures. Lust and limerence can be infused and enriched into your relationship at any point, but it isn't the default drive for most people years into a relationship, and it requires more effort than it did at the start of your relationship. But herein lies the trouble: Comfort and safety can render complacency. And complacency can lead us to take the magic of effort for granted.

CASE STUDY

Parker and her partner, Rori, had been dating for two years. Neither of them wanted children or to be married, but they decided to try living together and building a life as DINKs (Dual Income No Kids). They both had nieces and nephews, and felt grateful to have some young people in their world, and then equally grateful to get back to their lives. Living in NYC, there were always things to do, and their lives were full. Moving in together would streamline some of their chaos, reducing their commutes to one another and giving them more time to be together without having to go out. Both Rori and Parker worked from home, and initially, the move-in was great. They cooked together, picked out furniture, hosted dinner parties, and traveled together for about two years. In that time, they had sex often and everywhere in their apartment, exploring some kink and even obtaining a sex swing. But after about two years, they both noticed a decline in their sex lives and desire. More and more, time that had been dedicated to sexual intimacy was spent in athleisure wear on the couch. They both wanted a return to their hot sex life, but were struggling to build intimacy back into their days. It was easier to wind down each day with takeout and the latest episode of whatever series they were watching, than it was to muster up the energy to make out. Nothing bad had happened in their relationship; they both felt secure and loving with each other. In fact, Parker had never felt so safe. But their de-prioritization of sex had become alarming. After about three months they both wondered, have we stopped being lovers and become roommates?

Is It Normal to Feel Like Roommates?

Nearly all long-term relationships have phases where romance and sexuality take a back seat. Signaling a level of comfort and stability, partners in a roommate phase may feel secure enough to focus on other priorities for a while. Sharing household chores, financial obligations, and other experiences of daily living can be pragmatic and navigating these tasks together can strengthen trust, collaboration, and friendship between partners. A strong bond, shared history, and mutual respect can foster deep emotional intimacy in this phase, even if lust has taken a back seat. Temporary life circumstances may feel at the top of the priority list for one or both partners, serving as a distraction to sexual desire. The roommate phase is often temporary; there is no set time or duration that is healthy or unhealthy. How long partners stay in this phase depends on how much they prioritize sex, if they address any external factors, and when they decide it's time to invest energy into the erotic.

How Do We Get Out of the Roommate Phase?

It isn't always easy to get out of the roommate phase. In the case of my partner and I, we had discussed our sex life many times. Both of us agreed we wanted to get back to a place where intimacy was a priority. We discussed our needs and obstacles many times, to no avail. It had been three years of sexual mediocrity and we'd slipped into more of a platonic relationship. We were both living in resentment and it was taking a toll on our emotional connection. I expressed a desire for him to initiate something sexual or romantic and he didn't follow through. He felt pressure and wanted me to initiate an erotic scene, but I couldn't. I'd stopped seeing him as an erotic or sexual being. It had been so long, and while I loved him, I saw him as more of a friend or roommate.

This stalemate is common as rejection, disconnection, and outside stressors eat away at one or both partner's willingness to lean into a shift. For many couples, it can even become an unconscious power struggle—waiting to see who gives in first. Gone unresolved too long, the roommate phase can lead to a permanent change in how you see each other, transitioning your romantic relationship into a platonic one or pushing both of you onto separate paths. Consistent and mutual effort is often required to come back from this place, and if you're not on the same page when it comes to stoking the flames, it can further the divide between you and make it all the more challenging to find a path to sexual connection.

If you're like me and you've been waiting for your partner to initiate sex and get the ball rolling, but they can't or won't, here are some things you can do (and may have already tried) to be more assertive without directly initiating sex.

Consider how you've shared your feelings. Are you nonconfrontational, supportive, and nonjudgmental? Or has your frustration leaked all over the conversation? Use "I" statements, make requests, and discuss the impact on you, instead of placing blame on your partner.

Get curious about their perspective. Ask your partner questions in earnest to better understand what might be going on for them. Perhaps there are stressors, physical or mental health concerns, or performance fears getting in the way of their willingness to initiate. Try to understand where they're coming from, so you can look for solutions collaboratively.

Clarify your expectations. Gain clarity on each other's hopes, desires, and needs related to sexual intimacy. It's possible they've changed, and perhaps one or both of you want something now that you didn't before. Watch out for entitlement: Sex is not a given. Defining your expectations can be a starting point for transparency and renegotiation.

Rule out serious issues. Be honest with each other about whether there are bigger concerns, such as a health scare or mental health concern, or a rupture in the relationship that hasn't been discussed or remains unresolved. Work together to ensure these issues are not ignored and that you are genuinely satisfied with the relationship otherwise.

Collaborate toward a sustainable solution. Instead of relying on your partner to initiate sex, consider the benefit of taking the lead. Perhaps you can agree to alternate invitations, releasing some of the pressure from one partner to get sex going.

Increase nonsexual physical affection. For some partners, non-sexual intimacy begins to fade (or has already faded) when sexual intimacy starts to wane. Infusing your partnership with consensual, nonsexual touch can get you back in the habit of appreciating each other's physical touch.

Build a deeper emotional connection. A strong emotional connection is often a key ingredient in long-term sexual satisfaction. Partners who invest in intellectual, emotional, and spiritual intimacy often have an easier path back to sexual intimacy. Commit to rediscovering each other every day and consider how the novelty of seeing each other in new ways can add psychological space and eroticism.

Work with a sex therapist. If you've tried these steps and remain locked in a platonic plateau, but want to rekindle romance and sexual connection, working with a sex therapist may be the next step to help you get unstuck.

The roommate phase becomes problematic when one or both partners stop wanting to put in effort or start neglecting each other romantically or emotionally. Lingering ruptures in the relationship, coupled with ineffective solutions or avoidance, can set you adrift beyond the sexual sphere and result in a waning connection.

What If We're Too Close?

In the attachment or roommate phase, what is familiar often starts to feel familial. This is especially true when you live and/or have kids together. Further entrenching the confusion is a lack of sufficient boundaries: emotional, physical, or sexual. This can be understood as a form of enmeshment, and it looks like diffuse boundaries (unclear and undefined) with little differentiation between where one person stops and the other begins. Our partners become proxies for our attachment needs and projections. Unaddressed trauma or relational patterns become loud during this stage of your relationship.

As highlighted earlier in this chapter, some element of psychological (and sometimes physical) space is often a requirement for eroticism. A lack of psychological space can feel too close, engulfing, suffocating, and entrapping. This is not an ideal jumping-off point when it comes to sex. Enmeshment between partners can complicate desire and the question of compatibility, as it can lead to desexualization in an effort to avoid being totally consumed or overwhelmed. It may not make conscious sense, but to the unconscious mind, space is taken where it can be taken by removing sex from the equation.

On top of that, for partners who were raised by enmeshed parents, their psychological identity can suffer in development. In an enmeshed family system, individuality and individuation are not tolerated well. When enmeshment—sometimes called "covert incest" or "emotional incest"—has been unexplored and unaddressed, the pattern of behavior begins to repeat and take place in romantic relationships. This will look like a lack of boundaries between partners with very little space for differentiation. For many adult children of enmeshed parents, it is difficult to be loving and sexual with the same person if they had a parent who consciously or unconsciously required them to carry the load of their feelings. Enmeshed parents rarely do this with conscious intention; rather, they do not have sufficient skills or resources to attend to their own emotional needs, so they rely, inappropriately, on their children to engage in adult-like attunement to them.

In the case of covert incest, this is even trickier, because in a parent–child relationship where there has been some erotic charge, a parent might have put an emotional burden on their child that should have gone to their partner. Other examples of covert incest include having a parent who sexualized the child's body, discussed details of their own sex life with their child, or demanded to have details about their child's romantic or sexual experiences. Separate from sexual abuse or incest, covert incest does not involve sexual contact from a parent to a child. If one or both adult partners experienced enmeshment growing up, they may not have adequate boundaries in place to protect their partnership. Blurred boundaries and closer attachment can lead to an unconscious need for self-protection, driven to ensure they do not get engulfed in the partnership. The partner becomes a proxy for the enmeshed parent, and the enmeshed adult child unconsciously keeps the partner at a distance. This is often a misplaced boundary, as it may not feel emotionally safe to have boundaries with the enmeshed parent (even if they are estranged or deceased).

If you or your partner remains enmeshed with a parent as an adult, there may not be any space for sex with your partner as your parent may still be getting your prioritized (nonsexual) attention. Inappropriate loyalties to a parent threaten an adult child's sense of self and independence, leaving them more fiercely protective of their energy and investment with romantic partners.

Am I Settling?

A common fear is that you are letting go of better opportunities by staying with your current partner. But what if it's not all bad and there are elements of the relationship that you appreciate and enjoy? It can be tough to discern what is realistic when evaluating for FOMO versus looking at true compatibility. What are your priorities in partnerships? One person's settling is another person's dream relationship, so try not to compare you and your partner with the glossy veneer you see depicted of other peoples' relationships. A good place to start is to differentiate between what feels comfortable and what's missing. Comfort is a goal in partnership, but settling involves compromising on essential needs and desires—those that you've determined are paramount to your happiness. Staying in a relationship where your most prioritized needs and desires are consistently unmet is likely to lead to resentment, relationship dissatisfaction, and a decrease in overall happiness.

Not sure if you're settling? Notice the red flags. If you're settling, you're likely to notice ongoing resentment toward your partner, feelings of discontent, or feeling perpetually unfulfilled. You may want to reevaluate your relationship more closely. Are you experiencing reciprocated effort from your partner, or do you feel like you're carrying the relationship? Do you have healthy and productive conversations about where either of you feels amiss? Or do your conversations quickly devolve without empathy or resolution? Are you fantasizing about what life would be like if you left? Are you feeling held back? Have you communicated these concerns to your partner, only to have them remain overlooked or minimized? If you said yes to any of these red flags, it may be time to reevaluate whether this relationship is still a good fit for you. People change, you and your partner included.

Should I Stay or Should I Go?

Deciding you want to leave a relationship can be scary and can bring up specific fears. Concern about being alone or having regrets can leave people stuck in their unhappiness, but also not sure if they can be OK on their own. It can be hard to end a partnership when you love someone, even though you are unhappy. It can be hard to leave even if you *don't* love them like that anymore. Fear of judgment, failure, confrontation, stigma, or hurting your partner can make your unhappiness in the relationship seem like the path easier traveled.

Staying in a relationship that no longer fits can also bring with it significant concerns. Not having the kind of relationship or sex that is fulfilling takes a toll on your long-term health and well-being. Asking yourself the following questions can help you decide which path is the better of the two, or the lesser of two evils.

- Am I staying in this less sexually satisfying relationship because I'm afraid to be alone or afraid I won't find someone else?

- Am I engaging in martyrdom and sacrificing my own sexual satisfaction and exploration to avoid hurting my partner (or our family/children)?

- Am I avoiding these conversations with my partner due to a fear of what the confrontation may bring? Do I feel safe?

- Am I afraid I'm making the wrong choice, and will regret leaving this person I love and otherwise feel comfortable with, or am I unsatisfied in more than just the sexual domain of our relationship?

Ultimately, only you can decide what is best for you. There is risk in leaving, but there is also the possibility of a positive change. There is also a risk in staying in a relationship that leaves you feeling underwhelmed or undiscovered. What are the costs on your well-being, and on your children (if you have them), if nothing changes? What do you have to make peace with to stay?

Pleasure Points

- Long-term relationships go through predictable phases, driven by different human drives: lust, connection, and attachment.

- It is common to have a roommate phase (or several) across the lifespan of your relationship.

- A history or current practice of enmeshment or a lack of boundaries can lead to desexualization in relationships.

- Assessing whether you are settling and would be better off leaving a relationship comes down to recognizing ongoing resentment, lack of fulfillment, and being honest with yourself about the kinds of risk you're willing to take, whether to stay or leave.

Pleasure Reflections

- Are you in a rut or a roommate phase? How have you gone about bringing this up with your partner?

- Have you noticed any signs of psychological or emotional enmeshment, either when growing up or with your partner? How has that influenced your relationship with desire?

- When you think about staying in this relationship, what gives you comfort that it's the right decision? What scares you?

Part 3

What Can I Do About It?

Reclaiming desire is not as easy as flipping a switch or taking a pill. The first two sections in this book examine several of the most common obstacles to desire, but you may be wondering what to do now that you've identified the ones getting in your way. Naming the issue is one thing; solving it is another.

In this section, each chapter covers one of the various aspects of getting reconnected: to yourself, to a partner, to your body, and to pleasure. Decentering sex and centering a return to yourself may paradoxically be the most important step in reestablishing an erotically fulfilled life. Everyone's reclamation looks a little different, so try not to impose a rigid plan on yourself. Here are a few steps to consider along the way.

Chapter 13

What Actually Turns Me On?

It became very clear to me early in my career that many people don't know what turns them on and that they believe this is a problem. I'd ask questions in therapy with individuals or couples about what excites them or what they want to try, and sometimes the answers are clear and fast. But it's just as common for clients to look at me blankly or through eyes filled with shame or bewilderment, and utter, "I don't know."

You may feel this is a weakness, but I see it as an opportunity. You don't have to know what turns you on to have great sex. Sure, it can help to have some ideas, and if you are already clear on what turns you on, that's great. But not knowing can set the stage for exploring what you find erotic, and that, for many people, is what's hot. In fact, even if you already have a clear idea of what revs your desire, being open to exploration can keep you in a state of sexual wonder.

Expectations about pleasure from sex can inhibit a willingness to be curious and venture into the unknown. I'm not suggesting you have to enjoy or do things that do not interest you, but to instead reflect on what limiting expectations you may have internalized about sex that could be eclipsing your desire or pleasure. Consider if any of the following thoughts have crossed your mind.

I have to like what's normal.

There is no such thing as "normal" when it comes to sex. Assuming you must like what's "normal" can lead to self-censorship, self-abandonment, and a loss of desire. Fearing the judgment of others is a real desire killer.

I should always be spontaneously in the mood.

Spontaneous desire is not a sustainable standard, and the reality of desire is that it often depends on the context. By default, we feel desire as a response to something. Expecting yourself to feel desire spontaneously can apply pressure and create anxiety in your sexual exploration, which can inhibit curiosity and an authentic experience.

My partner should know what I want or like instinctively.

Assuming a partner should know what you like, or lead you to what you like, can result in resentment, frustration, and unmet expectations for both of you. Even if your partner has a general idea about what turns you on, it is your responsibility to be open about what you like and to advocate for your own pleasure, especially if you and your partner are not on the same page.

I have to look a certain way to be considered desirable.

Believing you are only worthy of receiving desire or pleasure if you look a certain way is a form of deprivation baked into patriarchal culture. Patriarchy tells women to conform to a certain aesthetic or run the risk of not being chosen or protected by the group and can be a precursor to sexual shut down.

I have to have an orgasm for it to count as good sex.

Excessive emphasis on having orgasms as the sole marker of good sex is a recipe for bad sex. When you overemphasize the need for an orgasm, it creates pressure between partners, often leading to frustration and performative behavior. Instead, focus on the multitude of sensations and emotions you feel during sex. Focus on pleasure.

Sex needs to be perfect every time.

What does perfect even mean? Expecting a sexual experience to be without any hiccups or awkward moments can perpetuate anxiety, shame, and disappointment, and in doing so, erase your humanity. If there are imperfect moments, or sex feels unsatisfying or painful, consider this an opportunity to learn more about yourself or a partner.

I have to be equally interested in every aspect of sex.

Don't expect yourself to like all aspects of sex the same, as this ignores your individuality and requires changing emotional states and preferences. Give yourself room to be creative and to like some things more than others.

I have to fulfill a certain role or image as a partner.

If you genuinely like elements of sex that are ascribed to a gender or societal-based role, that's great. Feel free to keep incorporating those elements into your sex play. However, expecting yourself to conform to societal expectations can limit your authentic expression and pleasure potential.

My fantasies are too much.

Believing that what you like is outside of what is acceptable, either in frequency, theme or intensity, is another grift of the patriarchy that demands women stay small so they do not fully tap into their power and agency.

I shouldn't have to use toys or accessories to get off.

Sex toys and accessories have existed since the early ages, and wanting or needing them to source pleasure does not indicate a problem with you or your anatomy. In fact, it can be a celebration of sexual creativity!

I don't have the body to try that.

Every single body is worthy of pleasure. Your body does not need to be perfect (what is "perfect" anyway?) to like certain kinds of pleasure sensations, want to try different positions (as long as they are accessible), or to try accessories. If loving your body is difficult, aiming for body neutrality can help you move beyond this block in exploring what you like. In other words, even if you can't get to a place of body appreciation or body positivity, you can aim for nonjudgment.

Fantasies

Sex is a form of play, and for many adults, it's one of the only or most important forms of play. Just as when you were a child and could spend countless hours enjoying a story of make believe, sexual fantasies in adulthood offer a different kind of adventure. Not only can fantasies serve as a powerful enhancement for sexual pleasure, but they give us a medium to explore and engage in scenarios that may not be accessible in real life. The fact that they are imaginary is one of the reasons fantasies can hold so much amplifying charge in the emotional and physiological responses to pleasure.

A key liberating element of fantasies is that they never have to happen in real life. That is what makes them a safe place to explore various feelings, sensations, and emotions. Often, when a fantasy is brought into real life and played out, it is disappointing. Why? Because it stops being a projection and includes all of the real-life variables that make it less shiny or exciting. This is one reason porn and erotica are so popular. They give way to an imaginary place that is never contaminated by reality.

CASE STUDY

Miranda was shy to discuss her fantasies when asked about it in session. She had shared her interests with a few partners, and some did not react well. In fact, one man left their date early, citing some work project he forgot about that was suddenly due. She feared that her fantasies made her weird, promiscuous, or too much. Asked if she was interested in discussing them, she paused and quietly said she was ready. Speaking softly, she shared that a few years ago, she'd stumbled on a former partner's favorite porn site when she borrowed his computer. Curious, she looked through his history and found several videos featuring double vaginal penetration. She had never seen this visual before and was fascinated and confused. Didn't it hurt? Was it safe? What did it feel like?

Miranda began watching double penetration porn regularly and was surprised to find herself turned on. What did this mean about her? She couldn't reconcile the idea of two penises inside her vagina or anus, imagining it would be painful, messy, and super awkward in real life. But it was now the mainstay of her fantasies, and she wasn't sure why. With some exploration, she discovered that part of what felt so exciting about this idea was that two straight (in her fantasy) men would be so enamored by her—and so consumed with their desire for her—that they would be willing to touch their bodies and penises together just to be close to her.

With time, she began exploring this fantasy during solo sex with the use of multiple dildos and discovered the physical sensation was less interesting to her than the fantasy, so she decided not to invite this fantasy into reality. But after she had been with a new partner for a while, she did ask him to use a dildo in her anus while penetrating her vagina, and found that sensation combined with her fantasies (which he was open to incorporating into their sex play together) was a winning balance of the real and make-believe.

The gap between fantasy and reality can cause a loss of desire. When we fear awkwardness or a lack of safety in real life, it can be useful to home in on what it is you are actually trying to feel. Is it an emotion? Or a sensation? Or both? What is it that is *really, really* interesting? Is there a way to indulge in that without the element that is awkward?

Denying one's fantasies is a path to sexual grief and disconnection. Exploring them can take a lifetime. If you find yourself denying a fantasy because you're interpreting it as a quality of your character, please stop. Sometimes they can give us a window of understanding into some aspect of ourselves that is unexpressed or explored, but having a fantasy is just that—it's a fantasy. It's play. It's expression.

Many feminist colleagues in my practice have wondered aloud whether it is anti-feminist to enjoy fantasies of forced arousal or consensual non-consent. It's a fair question given the long history of patriarchal oppression that has led to countless acts of sexual violence, exploitation, and subjugation. However, forced arousal remains one of the top fantasies for women and femme folks, including those who identify as feminists. This is because the taboo is subversive. Fantasies are transgressive and give us space to explore different parts of our-selves, and even for those who fight against social injustice all day in their work, the idea of leaning into the fear can be powerful. Fantasies are not real. Just because you have a fantasy that involves a breach in consent or aggressive physical activity does not mean you want those things to happen in real life—to you or anyone else. What makes the feeling so exciting is the knowledge and comfort of being in control. Paradoxically, even fantasies about being out of control are about be-ing *in* control. A fantasy ends whenever you stop and is guided only by you. You are always in control of a fantasy, so you can play with feelings that may not otherwise feel safe to explore.

Sensory Play

Not everyone is into fantasies or the emotional and cognitive as-pects of pleasure. For some, the sensory realm is their playground. Stimulating various senses is a surefire way to feel more pleasure and learn about what you like. Sensory play can be creative, experimen-tal, novel, and exciting. It can create bonding opportunities between partners as it offers a context for the giving and receiving of feedback in real time, allowing you to practice attunement with each other. Perhaps most importantly, sensory play fosters a space for you to de-velop and strengthen interoception—an awareness of internal sen-sations—reinforcing an embodied sense of play. Not sure where to start? You probably already have access to some accessories at home that can amplify your sexual pleasure and don't cost much at all. Here are a few low or no-cost ways to play with different sensations.

- Blindfolds: Limiting your sight may not feel like sensory play, since it inhibits one of your senses, but it enhances your other senses and builds anticipation. You don't have to have a formal blindfold, instead you can substitute things around the house like a scarf, soft sleep mask, tea towel, or even a T-shirt. Just ensure you like the way the fabric feels against your skin and that it's comfortable.

- Feather ticklers: Feathers can provide a host of sensations and can be a great way to build up sensory tease in touch. If you don't want to spend a lot of money on a fancy tickler, you can buy different kinds of feathers at a craft store or use a clean (unused) feather duster.

- Warm and cold textures: Experimenting with temperature play can be a titillating compilation of contrasts. For easy props, try some ice cubes, freezable facial rollers, or cool metal objects on your skin, or skin-safe wax, warm towels (wet or dry for additional sensation play), or melted chocolate or caramel chips. It's best to keep these products on the skin and avoid penetration to avoid the risk of infections.

- Scented candles or essential oils: The olfactory system is a major player in the game of arousal, so find some scents that arouse and excite you. You can incorporate them directly (like the scent of your lover's cologne or sweat) or create ambience with scent in your sexual space. Stock up on candles, essential oil diffusers, or massage oils that bring an aromatic addition to the experience. If you like the smell of your partner, perhaps even throw on one of their slightly worn T-shirts to keep them present in a steamy solo sex session.

- Fabrics: Experiment with different textures on your skin, like a soft silky scarf, faux fur blanket, or soft flannel sheet. Perhaps you like something a little more intense—grab a wool blanket or scratchy pillow to serve as a kind of scratching post.

- Edible treats: Incorporating foods and edible accessories can really enhance your taste and touch. You can use all kinds of foods; syrups, jams, whipped cream, honey, or even flavored lubes or arousal serums.

- Massage and pressure tools: Sensual massages or pressure play can help relax tension and heighten tactile sensations. Experiment with different pressures, speeds, and tactile options. Easy go-to props around the house can include a rolling pin to roll on the skin, a plastic pie crust scalloping tool, silicone gloves, soft bristle brushes, or plastic or metal baking tools for a light scratching sensation. Pro tip: Don't use the same tools for cooking and sex! If you do, make sure they've been well sanitized before and after each use.

- Music and ambient sounds: Implement an aural background that is relaxing or rhythmic in a way that compliments how you like to move your body to enhance your sense of embodiment and context. Many streaming services have built-in playlists or the ability to create your own, or you can use nature sounds, brown noise, or other kinds of ambient sound that take you to another level. Experiment with different styles of music. Do you like music with lyrics or without? What about music from different cultures or areas of the world, or music that taps into certain emotions?

Whatever kind of sensory experience you want to explore, remember to communicate with your partner (if you're playing with them) to explore how they experience it, too. If you feel uncomfortable communicating your desires, you can always start your sensory exploration during solo sex to get a better sense of what you like without the influence of another person.

Am I Vanilla or Kinky?

The spectrum of sexual pleasure is vast, and the line between vanilla and kinky can be blurry as more and more activities that were once considered completely taboo have come into the mainstream. "Vanilla sex" is a term used to describe conventional or traditional

sexual activities that are considered standard, including intimate activities like kissing, touching, oral sex, and penetrative intercourse
without the addition of role playing, bondage, or power dynamics.

Vanilla sex is often aligned with the idea of romance and can be
more focused on connection and intimacy between partners. For
many people, it is more accessible and approachable and does not
require a lot of extra effort or additional mental load that can come
with kinkier or less conventional contexts. It can be lower pressure,
may require less physical or emotional effort, and can be adapted
to suit a wide variety of comfort levels, positions, and locations. In
that sense, it is often straightforward when it comes to discussing
desires, boundaries, and preferences, whereas kinkier sex is more
nuanced with complex sexual scenes, making vanilla sex safer and
easier for people to enjoy on a regular basis.

Some people like to dabble in kink to augment a generally vanilla
preference in their sex lives, and others need kinkier practices to feel
aroused. Whether or not you like kink doesn't say anything about
your character. Pleasure is a complex experience, comprising our beliefs, emotions, and physical sensations and the meaning we attach
to them. Because kink often involves activities that are considered
taboo, its sometimes transgressive nature can be a part of someone's personal empowerment, bucking norms and resisting sexual
repression, and foraging a space for personal growth. Some people
find immense empowerment in dynamics that play with power, such
as BDSM, as the consensual and controlled space gives way to the
exploration of holding or relinquishing power through dominant or
submissive roles.

Kink can be healing in the aftermath of trauma or oppression, as
it focuses on mutuality, consent, and communication. Engaging in
transgressive or subversive sexual activities can help people reframe

their own personal narrative around events in their lives where they didn't have control. This sexual storytelling can be an essential element of personal self-discovery, identity formation, and relationship building. Kink, after all, is more about intimacy than it is about sex. It gives partners a playful way to strengthen their communication and negotiation skills and practice consent, attunement, aftercare, and debriefing. This can also happen in vanilla encounters, but the practice of conscious kink builds in steps to ensure comfort, communication, and ongoing consent, like discussing interests, limits, and aftercare needs, negotiating what will take place during a scene, playing out the scene, and then participating in intentional aftercare and debriefing. The focus on clear communication and respect for boundaries can be a necessary and positive contrast to societal narratives that often lack clarity around power and mutuality.

Kink can build trust and intimacy. It emphasizes being vulnerable (when assuming new roles or playing with intense sensations) and exploring each other's desires and boundaries. The possibilities within kink are limitless, offering ongoing variety and novelty to prevent monotony in the bedroom. Each play scene is something you can customize to your mood and needs in that moment. Also, the intensity of play, sensation, or endorphins in kink can lead to altered states of consciousness that are euphoric or trance-like. Many kinksters find respite and belonging in the greater kink community as a place where they can be accepted, supported, and educated in their sexual preferences. For many, kink is not just something they do, it's who they are, and the community is a kind of chosen family, even when there are no sexual activities involved.

Not sure if you're more kinky or more vanilla? You don't have to be one or the other, and neither is better or worse for desire as a whole. Try to move away from qualifying vanilla sex or kinky sex as better or worse. Remember, human beings are diverse and so are their sexual preferences. Whichever you prefer, having the sex you like makes it super-hot. It's not about what you're doing, it's about how you are feeling. So, don't let anyone else yuck your yum, and don't judge yourself for what you like. There is no hierarchy of hot sex, only subjective enjoyment. If it works for you and is consensual, that is all that matters.

Are Your Desires Prescribed or Chosen?

One of the trickiest ideas that can thwart desire and pleasure is that there is one prescribed way to be in order to be healthy or valid. Take, for example, monogamy. Sold and packaged to us as *the way things are* in films, stories, and literature, the push for monogamy as the only healthy choice for relationships is a lie. Relationship orientations ranging from monogamy to nonmonogamy to relationship anarchy (a romantic relationship that does not fit any rules or expectations) can all be healthy or unhealthy depending on how they are carried out. There is certainly no shortage of monogamous relationships waylaid by infidelity and deception. As a result, many sex therapists understand that the social pressures leading to compulsory monogamy can impede desire, pleasure, and overall satisfaction.

Compulsory monogamy is like a costume we put on for a role we are playing on the stage of social expectation. The script is written by alleged tradition rather than personal desire or interest. External pressures from family, friends, or cultural norms dictate our choice of relationship as the only valid form of partnership.

Intentional monogamy, in contrast, factors in personal agency, deliberate choice, and authenticity unconstrained by social expectations or predetermined relationship narratives. Intentional monogamy is about recognizing that other relationship constellations are equally healthy and valid, and choosing monogamy may be the best for you, given your personal desires, preferences, and values. It's a dance of mutual consent, as opposed to a forced conclusion and trajectory. Partners actively communicate, negotiate, and set the terms for their monogamous relationship fluidly, giving space for individual expression and the cocreation of a relationship dynamic that is unique to them.

As you reflect on your own feelings about monogamy, consider the following questions to unmask the layers of influence from society, religion, and pop culture, to discern whether you are following a path of compulsory or intentional monogamy (if you are monogamous).

- What are the origins of your expectations about monogamy? Are they shaped by a desire to conform or your authentic relational needs and desires?

- Is monogamy your default setting? Have you considered alternative relationship structures and actively chosen monogamy to be the best fit from a place of agency, not a place of fear?

- Assess your communication about monogamy with your partner. Have you openly discussed your mutual desires, relational expectations, and boundaries or have you assumed them as an expected path for a monogamous relationship?

- Have you considered the pros and cons of monogamy, as well as the advantages and disadvantages of nonmonogamy? Does it feel off-limits to even entertain that question?

- Are you and your partner open to renegotiating the terms of your relationship, exploring new possibilities, and adapting to each other's changing needs or circumstances?

- What brings you fulfillment in monogamy? Is this in line with your authentic relational needs? Or are the aspects you like about monogamy more aligned with your need to be perceived a certain way?

The purpose of these questions is not to encourage you to be nonmonogamous if that doesn't fit you. It is to help you question paradigms that may be stifling your desire, autonomy, and pleasure. Because monogamy has been touted as the "normal" path of relationships, people who have a different relationship orientation can often find themselves suppressed in obligatory monogamous relationships and are woefully unhappy. Conversely, for some people, monogamy gives them the most peace and contentment. Neither of these options is inherently right or wrong, better or worse, so give yourself permission to be intentional about what feels right for you.

Similarly, heterosexuality is often erroneously viewed as the default sexual orientation rather than as a mode of reproduction within a patriarchy,[1] with same-sex relationships and pleasure wrongfully seen as an irregularity. While procreation may require opposite biological contributions, pleasure does not. Much in the same way society has pushed a narrative of monogamy as the expected path, so has it pushed a narrative of heterosexuality. Many women partner and have had sex only with men due to the subtle force of compulsory heterosexuality, or "comphet" for short. Comphet is a script handed down to many women before they even learn to write their own narrative, with parents assuming their gender and sexuality even in utero, and making statements and assumptions about their future partners and their romantic and sexual destiny. These assumptions (of parents and society) nudge us toward a predetermined destination, often without conscious consideration. Comphet assumes heterosexuality is the default orientation, and anything else requires a coming out or a justification. All sexual orientations are natural and healthy, and a default. Humans are diverse, and procreation is not the only reason for sex or pleasure, despite what patriarchal scripts may want us to believe. There is nothing wrong with heterosexuality, and again, it is not the intention of this book to convince you that your sexual orientation needs to be examined or changed. It doesn't. If, however, you've arrived at an understanding of your sexual orientation that reflects an obligatory path and does not align with your authentic desires, you can give yourself permission to step onto a different path. If you find yourself frequently wondering about or desiring a path where attractions may transcend the binaries of gender or sexuality, but find yourself limited to narrow and obligatory boxes, perhaps you have been performing straightness and denying a part of yourself that is more expansive. Consider these questions to discern between compulsory heterosexuality or sexual fluidity.

- Reflect on your sexual desires. Are they shaped by your authentic identity and guided without suppression, or are you limiting yourself and your desires out of fear or a sense of duty to a script?

- Have you ever allowed yourself to consider expanded views of attraction?

- Have you noticed shifts or changes in who or what you desire over different periods of your life?

- Are you feeling pressure to conform to heteronormative scripts for your family, your career, or to avoid negative social repercussions?

- Do the narratives woven by your attractions align with your true desires or are they formed and restricted by what has been labeled socially acceptable?

- Do you feel anchored to a fixed sexual orientation and devoid of authentic desire?

- Have you never considered other options because being in a heterosexual relationship is *just what you do*?

The opposite of compulsory heterosexuality is not a different sexual orientation. In fact, you may decide that you are decidedly straight and that is OK! The opposite of comphet is sexual liberation and sexual autonomy. It is freedom. It is choice. Liberation is sexy. Liberation is pleasure.

Drop the Need for Perfection

When considering what really turns you on, remember to minimize the things that turn you off. In this case, the need for perfection. As noted in chapter 5, perfectionism is a strategy to avoid shame. One of the best ways to learn more about what really turns you on is to leave room for the messiness and humanness of sex and life. In good sex, your body will make noises, your skin may reflect dimples or stretch marks, there will likely be fluids and sometimes even smells. You may make goofy faces or breathe in a way that confuses you with a feral animal. Good. Make noise if you want to make noise, but not because it's expected of you. Drop the performance and the spectating and just be yourself. Sex is messy and imperfect and so is everyone.

Pleasure Points

- Embrace the reality that you may not know what turns you on. The opportunity in that is an unfolding of erotic exploration.

- Limiting expectations can hinder pleasure and the inquiry about what really turns you on. Abandon the expectation of conformity and pursue authentic curiosity and enjoyable sensations.

- Recognize sexual fantasies as a form of play and an avenue for self-exploration and expression, free from the burdens of real-life consequences.

- Sensory play is often a path of enhanced sensual and sexual pleasure. Give yourself permission to get creative.

- Whether you enjoy kinky sex, vanilla sex, or both, remember to appreciate the empowerment of cultivating a cache of sexual activities that you enjoy.

Pleasure Reflections

- What are my beliefs about monogamy and nonmonogamy? If I am monogamous, is my monogamy intentional or compulsory? How do my views about monogamy influence my desires?

- How has the idea of compulsory heterosexuality influenced my sexual orientation and my desires? Am I stifling my desires due to societal pressures?

- What, if any, limitations am I placing on my desires due to preconceived ideas about what sex should or should not be? How can I let go and make space for the messy and imperfect aspects of sex, so I can be sexual with more authenticity?

Chapter 14

What Are My Needs, Boundaries, and Values?

An integral step to improving your sex life is understanding what you like and why it's important to you (values), what parameters have to be in place for you feel safe, relaxed, and receptive to pleasure (needs), and what your limits are or what makes desire or arousal less possible for you (boundaries). You may already have a sense of your sexual values, needs, and boundaries, though it helps to define them explicitly if you're struggling to feel turned on. Expectations and social scripts are passed down to most of us, though we rarely stop to consider the consequences of those experiences.

CASE STUDY

Priya had a long list of shoulds and should-nots when it came to sex and she was feeling wildly unsatisfied in her sex life. She was not in a committed relationship and wanted to explore her sexuality, but she was nervous about the outcome, what casual partners might think of her, or what her family would say if they knew she was OK with having casual sex. When I asked her what *she* thought of herself for wanting to explore casual sex, she wasn't sure. She didn't judge other people for wanting casual sex, but something was holding her back. She never really thought about her own values around sex, and like many people, had unconsciously adopted the views of her family and culture.

Priya was ready to get curious with herself about what she valued sexually and where it contradicted her inherited values so that she could explore her options. She didn't even know how to get started in seeking casual sex partners. What would she tell them? Could she even expect to have a conversation with them before having sex? Priya had questions and felt ready to get clear on her needs and boundaries so she could be more prepared to self-advocate with partners.

There is not a rigid formula to figuring out what works for you, but in this chapter I'll offer you a framework to get started. You'll be able to adjust your approach as you learn more about your sexual intentions, as well as the accelerators and inhibitors of your desire. Keep in mind that every sexual opportunity and context is different because you are different in every situation. While there may be constants to your arousal, needs, or limits, it is important to stay flexible and make sure to account for your own dynamic states of being. Your sexual needs may change with different emotional states, different partners, different phases of life, or the changing experience of living in your body.

Outlining Your Sexual Values

Clarifying your sexual values can help you build a personal blueprint for erotic satisfaction and safety, so we'll start with an assessment. Think of it as a journey of self-discovery and healing that will also help you gain a precise understanding of what actually matters to you in your sexual experience. This reflection seeks to understand your authentic experience, which can lead to vulnerability with partners and foster coherence and integrity within yourself. When you are authentic, it increases a sense of safety with yourself and what you bring to a sexual encounter, and it can empower you to have healthier and more satisfying sexual experiences with others.

How do you start to examine the underpinnings of your beliefs and values about sex and intimacy? By getting introspective. For this exercise, get some paper or a journal to jot down your notes, or come back to it later when you have more time. Ask yourself the following questions on how they relate to your opinions about sex. Don't try to polish your answers, just start with your immediate responses. You can always revisit them later if there is a belief you'd like to challenge or think about differently.

- How do I prioritize and discuss consent in my sexual interactions? What allows me to feel safe and turned on in these discussions?
- In what ways would I like to be shown respect by a partner in sexual interactions?

- Is either physical pleasure or emotional intimacy more important to me or contingent on the other? Are they equally important to me? How would I like to balance physical pleasure with emotional intimacy?

- What does it look or feel like to be authentic in my sexual expression?

- How do I work to create equality and mutuality in my sexual relationships and experiences? (Even in kinky scenes where power imbalances are key, how do I create a foundation of equality to establish safety in the play?)

- How important is playfulness in my sexual experiences? What kinds of playfulness are welcome? What kinds of playfulness might be a distraction?

- What role do I want sexual fantasies to play in my overall satisfaction?

- How do I view diverse body types, including my own?

- How important are adventure and spontaneity to me sexually, during solo sex and with partners?

- How important is it to me to incorporate a spiritual or transcendent aspect to my sexuality? Why is this important to me?

- How important is nonsexual affection with partners? What does it communicate to me?

- How do I want to stay informed about my sexual health, partners' sexual health, or sex education in general?

- What allows me to feel safe enough in sexual experiences and what steps would I like to take to prioritize those needs?

- How do I establish and maintain mutuality in the prioritization of pleasure?

- What are my views about the intersection of sexuality and commitment in a relationship?

- How important is sexual pleasure in the overall picture of my holistic well-being?

- What social expectations and influence about sexuality am I most in agreement with? Which expectations do I disagree with? Why?

- What role does self-love, self-acceptance, and body image play in my sexual confidence?

- What, if any, cultural or religious influences shape my approach to sexuality?

- What sexual stigmas or shame am I consciously carrying? How would I like to challenge them? What fears are present at the idea of letting them go?

- What guides my preferences and approach to sexual exclusivity versus consensual nonmonogamy?

- How do I balance the needs for autonomy and space with my need for connection in my romantic and sexual relationships?

- What stereotypes about gender roles influence how I see myself and my relationship with sex? In what way do I agree with them or actively work to dismantle them?

- How do I want to learn from sexual experiences? What might I need from a partner in terms of aftercare or debriefing after a sexual experience? What would I like my personal practice of reflection to consist of?

- How do I handle challenges, conflicts, differences in preferences, or desire discrepancies with a partner? What are my deal-breakers?

- How important is it that my partner and I have shared sexual values? What significance do I attribute to the presence or absence of shared sexual values?

- How do I incorporate mindfulness and presence into my experience of pleasure? How would I like to practice sexual mindfulness alone and with partners?

- How do I feel about working with a sex therapist or other sexual health professional to address concerns I have about sexuality?

- How do I consciously work toward the construction of a sex-positive mindset or environment by myself? With partners? In the community?

This is not a definitive list, but it can get you started on an investigation into your sexual values. It's a starting point for other questions that may help you refine your opinions and beliefs. Having a better understanding of your sexual values is essential to becoming more aware of your needs for sexual pleasure. Everything from your sexual identity, sexual embodiment, needs, desires, and boundaries are all shaped by the core principles outlined by your sexual values.

Defining Your Needs

Your needs may be specific to a sexual moment, or they may extend to the nonsexual experiences you have with yourself and with partners. Consider this list of needs and make note of how you define them, what it would look like to have these needs met (and by whom), and which needs feel important to you and your current relationship with sex.[1]

acceptance	awareness	choice
acknowledgment	beauty	clarity
affection	belonging	closeness
appreciation	boundaries	collaboration
authenticity	celebration	communication
autonomy	challenge	companionship

competence

consciousness

consideration

consistency

contribution

cooperation

creativity

ease

efficacy

emotional
 connection

empathy

equality

exercise

exploration

food

freedom

growth

honesty

hope

humor

inclusion

independence

inspiration

integrity

intimacy

joy

learning

leisure

love

meaning

mourning

movement

mutuality

non-sexual touch

novelty

nurturance

organization

participation

peace

people

permission

play

pleasure

power

presence

purpose

respect

rest

safety

sensory activation

sexual expression

sexual touch

security

shelter

space

spiritual connection

spontaneity

stability

stimulation

to be heard

to be known

to be seen

to be understood

to hear

to know

to matter

to see

to understand

transparency

trust

understanding

warmth

water

Notice the reactions you had while considering this list of needs. What did you feel emotionally? What did you observe in your body? What needs stand out to you as immediate points of exploration? What needs do you meet for yourself? What needs do you struggle to meet for yourself? What needs do you feel comfortable expressing to a sexual or romantic partner? What needs leave you feeling vulnerable? What needs have been met well by partners? What needs, if any, feel perpetually unmet or under addressed? In reflecting on these needs, what might you add or change to any of your sexual values? What feels solidified?

There is no such thing as permanence in our state of being human, and as such, it's important to be in regular consultation with yourself about how your needs ebb and flow. Contrary to what we are sold as a promise of monogamy in media and social lore about relationships, it's completely unrealistic to expect one person or partner to meet all of your needs. If you're expecting a partner to fulfill your every whim and requirement, you may be setting yourself up for disappointment. Instead, try prioritizing your needs and think about which relationships in your life might be able to meet them. Some of your needs may be suitable for only a sexual partner to meet, while others can be met by friends, family, or other people in your life. Humans are community beings and it takes a village to support each of us.

How Will I Know It's Time to Reevaluate My Needs?

As your life unfolds and you collect experiences and perspectives, it's inevitable that your intrinsic needs, values, and boundaries will shift. You may start to feel discontent or a lack of fulfillment, which can signal that your needs have changed or that your approach to love or sex may be out of alignment. Once you feel that change, it's a good time to get curious about your internal states. Changes in your career, relationship status, family dynamics, growing children (if you have them), or health can redistribute what you find most important in life and in a relationship, both sexually and nonsexually.

Relationships are deeply intertwined with our needs. The quality of our closest relationships can evoke either tension or feelings of safety. Pay close attention to how you feel around your partner or others who are close to you and consider how changes in relationship dynamics may alter your core needs. Don't underestimate the power of a nonsexual relationship in your sexual fulfillment. For example, if your boss starts speaking down to you or giving you a hard time, you may seek out a sexual experience that is more tender or nurturing than you would otherwise.

A great indication that it's time to reexamine your current needs is when you feel exhausted or become aware that you have lost connection with a sense of purpose or passion in your life. If something that once brought you much joie de vivre now renders you without any internal momentum, it could indicate a change in your values or could be an indication of unmet needs. The same is true for feeling burned-out or overextended. If you're constantly feeling drained, you may need to advocate for different resources, learn to say no, and set different boundaries to better protect your energy and rebalance a sense of passion. This solution isn't always accessible when resources are limited or if you don't have allies who can pitch in.

As you continue to discover what you enjoy in sex and relationships or need to heal from other experiences in your life, you may also find yourself reconsidering your needs. Try to stay open to self-exploration and feedback from people you trust and who offer you constructive feedback as opposed to people committed to judging you. Feeling out of alignment with your needs or values can also take shape in a constant state of unease or discomfort around certain people, contexts, or things. Make note and don't minimize your body's cues of distress. Instead, you might pull out your list of needs and reconsider which ones are important to you in this context, and which needs are not being met well or at all.

Setting and Sustaining Boundaries

OK, so you have more clarity about your sexual and relational values and needs. Good! Now comes the fun—and sometimes very hard—part: setting boundaries that help people understand how best to be in relationship with you. In this exercise, you're invited to think about your romantic and sexual relationships, but you can apply these ideas to any kind of relationship: familial, platonic, professional, and so on.

What are boundaries? An assertion of boundaries is to communicate limits, express personal needs, seek consent, regulate emotions, and negotiate expectations in a relationship. Boundaries may be physical, emotional, sexual, financial, material, or spiritual. Similarly, when you evaluate the space between you and another person, you are able to assess safety and protection, definition of the self, accountability, empowerment, and mutual respect.

Despite how boundaries are often conveyed in the media, they do not serve as a tool to control other peoples' behavior. In fact, if you set boundaries hoping they will change how someone else acts toward you, you're likely to become embroiled in power struggles and disappointment galore. Boundaries are a guide for you to know what *you* will and will not tolerate with yourself or with others. Sharing your boundaries with another person gives them the opportunity to decide how they want to proceed with you, which in turn gives you important information about how you want to proceed with them or the relationship. It is best to let your boundaries be known and then observe how the other person responds. Do they respect your boundaries immediately? Do they question them, respectfully, to better understand you? Do they question your boundaries to under-mine and dismiss you? Do they bulldoze over your boundaries with-out concern? This is all essential information about your safety in a relationship.

Knowing your "yes" is an essential element of desire, but knowing your "no" is just as critical. You don't have to know all of your bound-aries ahead of setting them. Feeling your way into a boundary is of-ten how you begin to recognize what your limits might be and what allows you to feel most comfortable in a relationship. Sometimes it's best to experiment with a limit and pause for a moment to see if you might want to loosen a boundary or lean into a more protective stance. It's OK to change your mind and it's OK to have different boundaries with different people in different circumstances.

As mentioned earlier in regard to needs, if you're not sure how to begin evaluating your boundaries, start by noticing moments of discomfort in your interactions with others. Feeling uncomfortable is a key indication you have a need that is not being met. Your needs may become clearer by keeping your values in mind and balancing them with your body's cues about how you feel in the moment. From there, look at your needs and ask yourself, "What would satisfy this need? What must happen for it to feel met?"

CASE STUDY

Frances was thrilled to be dating a new partner, Chloe, and they were spending a lot of time together. Frances looked forward to their dates, but she noticed that Chloe was starting to hint that she'd like to spend more time together. Frances felt torn. She really liked Chloe and liked where this was going, but one of her core values around sex and dating was to not move too quickly. That means different things to different people, and for Frances, it meant not having more than two dates a week for the first three months she was dating someone. In past relationships, Frances went all in fast, and she lost herself in the process. Finding herself again after those relationships ended was painful, and she vowed to never over-prioritize an early relationship again, ensuring she kept some balance in her life.

As Chloe suggested more dates more frequently, Frances began feeling a heaviness in her chest and noticed that she started to feel dread whenever Chloe texted her. This was Frances's cue to determine what boundaries she would benefit from clarifying. She realized she never told Chloe about the plan she made with herself, so she took a risk and told her, "I really like you and our time together. In the past, I've struggled to prioritize myself when I really like someone, so I decided to commit to no more than two dates per week in the first three months. Is that something that can work for you?" Chloe was a little disappointed, but she understood and appreciated the transparency. It gave her security because she was starting to think Frances wasn't into her anymore, since she had started to feel her pull back.

What boundaries are you already good at setting and maintaining? Where do you struggle?

Here are some examples of boundaries in practice.

PHYSICAL BOUNDARIES

- "I need my own space for a little while each day so I can unwind, decompress, and chill out after work."

- "I haven't been sleeping well in our current arrangement. Let's discuss how we can approach our different sleeping preferences collaboratively, to accommodate both of our needs."

- "I don't feel comfortable with unexpected touch. I prefer that you check in with me before you touch me."

EMOTIONAL BOUNDARIES

- "I want to be supportive, but I am not open to taking responsibility for each other's feelings."

- "I'd like us to agree not to bring up each other's past mistakes during arguments, so we can stay focused on one issue at a time. Are you willing to commit to that?"

- "I need time to process my thoughts and feelings before we discuss a sensitive topic. I can be ready to have this conversation in an hour. Are you willing to revisit this after I've had a chance to get my thoughts together?"

FINANCIAL BOUNDARIES

- "I'd feel more comfortable with our collective spending if we agreed to a monthly budget."

- "I prefer to keep our money separate. Let's talk about how we can share expenses in a way that works for both of us."

- "It's important to me that we are transparent about money and savings for our future. I'm not comfortable not having a plan that feels equitable."

SEXUAL BOUNDARIES

- "Sex positivity is important to me. I need to be able to have a conversation about my desires that is free from judgment."

- "It seems that we like different things in bed. Let's set a time to discuss our sexual preferences so we can find some common ground."

- "I don't like when you initiate sex by grabbing at my genitals. Please stop."

SPIRITUAL BOUNDARIES

- "I really value my spiritual practice. Please don't mock it."
- "Let's agree that we have different spiritual beliefs and agree not to impose them on each other."
- "Let's explore how our spiritual beliefs align and how we can incorporate them into our daily lives together."

MATERIAL BOUNDARIES

- "Let's discuss how we can share responsibilities around the house equally to maintain fairness."
- "Respecting each other's belongings is a nonnegotiable for me. How can we ensure we maintain that respect?"
- "I'm not okay with you using my ___ without my explicit permission."

You may have noticed in reading these samples that some of them sound like a definitive and declarative boundary, letting the other person know what does not work for you. Some of the others express a need and the request that follows is more indirect, but it can be a softer launch into what could be a difficult conversation. Making a request of your partner to respect your boundary also reminds them of their volition and agency when choosing how to respond. Making a request that begins "Are you willing to . . ." specifically confronts their *willingness* and offers a moment of potential pause as they consider whether they are willing to meet your request, bolstering opportunities for individuality and accountability together. If someone

is not willing, it gives you a chance to get curious together about if
and how you can negotiate a middle ground.

Pleasure Points

- Understanding your sexual values, needs, and boundaries is
  essential in curating a thriving sex life.

- It is inevitable that your sexual needs, boundaries, and maybe
  even values will change over time. Revisit them as often as it
  feels right for you.

Pleasure Reflections

- How do you prioritize and communicate consent in your sexual
  interactions? What creates safety for you in these interactions?

- How would you like to show respect and be shown respect with
  partners in sexual interactions, given your needs for physical
  and emotional safety and pleasure?

- What boundaries, if any, might you be afraid to voice with
  partners? What fears are connected to these boundaries? How
  do you expect a partner to respond?

- What deal-breakers are you aware of during this chapter of
  your life?

Chapter 15

How Do I Get Back to My Body?

Sometimes, the first step to reclaiming or returning to your desire is getting back in touch with your body's sensations and felt experiences. But if you've been less connected to your body for a while, getting back into it can take some practice. It doesn't happen overnight—and disconnection or dissociation can repeat itself when you face increased stressors or triggers. With a regular practice of mindfulness and presence, you can reduce your sensitivity to some triggers over time and widen your window of tolerance, strengthening your capacity to feel without becoming dysregulated.

Feeling disembodied or not fully present can minimize painful feelings, but the cost is high. Muting or flattening intense emotions means positive emotions or sensations are also affected.

In order to feel pleasure, you have to be willing to risk feeling some pain. For some people, this is a zero-sum game. They're not interested. It's too much. It's good to know your limits and exercise them, but it's lonely and limiting to linger in such a restrictive place for too long. If you find yourself unable or unwilling to be guided by any of the exercises in this chapter, it might be an indication that you need assistance with deeper trauma work to develop your coping skills before you will feel safe enough to be in your body and find pleasure. While this chapter offers ideas on how you can safely practice embodiment, I trust your inner knowledge about your readiness or need for greater support. It is perfectly OK to start small and advance in incremental steps. Don't worry about what other people do as they go through the process of becoming more embodied, because there is no better or worse path through. Your timeline is yours. If anything I suggest feels too quick, feel free to slow it down. Spread it out. Take your time.

Conversely, if these exercises feel too slow and you feel compelled to rush through them, I invite you to slow yourself down or take a break. Often, people feel the urge to jump over the process of feeling to get to the end of the exercise. Fooled by the illusion that the exercise is "done," they have successfully bypassed mindfulness and have extended their own disconnection. That's not to say this approach is bad or wrong, but if you notice this pattern, perhaps slowing down or pausing to develop other coping skills might help you stay in the feelings with more ease.

Part of becoming embodied is being emotionally present. Some clinicians would say you don't have to be aware of your feelings to be embodied and others might say you don't have to be in your body to be emotionally present. I would say both statements are true-ish. Certainly, there are degrees of emotional and somatic presence that you can work on and develop separately, but there is inherent crossover given the integration of your mind and body.

Dissociation and numbness happen when the mind and body become compartmentalized, unable to communicate with ease and fluency. Beginning any practice of mindfulness or embodiment is to take a step toward integration. It can feel scary to begin healing in this way. This is why talk therapy is only so effective for healing trauma. The body keeps a record of memories, too, and at some point, the residue of earlier experiences needs to be explored somatically for integrated healing. That's not to say you can't feel heaps better with talk therapy, but many survivors frequently note that they finally feel free once they've had a healing experience that integrates the body.

Being emotionally present means fully engaging and connecting to your own emotions and/or the emotions of others in the here and now, without distraction, and demonstrating both empathy and compassion for yourself or someone else. It can be difficult to be present—which can look like active listening, acknowledging the emotion, being vulnerable and authentic in your feelings, and attuning to yourself or another person—when you're dysregulated. Attunement is another way of saying "tracking"—that is, following verbal or nonverbal cues, yours or someone else's.

If mindfulness is how we describe being present in one's mind, embodiment is how to manifest presence in your body. This entails developing interoception to better recognize physiological sensations, noticing shifts in your physiological states, and building awareness of the mind–body connection. Our brain and body are inextricably linked and are in a constant state of feedback. To be integrated and embodied means having access to the present experience of the mind, emotions, *and* body. Interoception (see chapter 5) is a key factor in building embodiment, as are exteroception and proprioception.* Each of these skills gives us different information about ourselves and the world, and how we interact in it. These are the building blocks of embodiment.

Creating a regular embodiment and mindfulness practice have been shown to reduce stress, since dysregulated emotions can keep the body in a chronically heightened state of nervous system arousal, increasing the allostatic load (damage caused by stress). Other benefits include improving immune function (due to the reduction in allostatic load), reducing muscle tension, reducing the risk of cardiovascular issues and digestive problems, improving sleep, improving conflict management, relational satisfaction, and of course, sexual desire.

How Do I Get Started?

There are different ways to explore embodiment: through sensory awareness, the navigation and manipulation of breath, and movement. You can practice all of these variations of embodiment on your own or with a partner. Practicing them with a partner shifts into what could be called conscious interaction or attunement. A common misconception for people who are just getting started is that they have to reinvent their whole day and suddenly live a 24-7 yoga life. Getting back into your body can include some more involved practices, but is often about the small things you can incorporate into your day without too much extra fuss, planning, or expense. Here is a short list of some exercises that have many variations, so you can find one that works for you.

---

* Exteroception is the perception of external stimuli from the environment around you through the five senses. Proprioception is the perception of your body's parts, their position and movement, relative to each other and the external environment. It is how you are able to walk through a door without bumping into the doorframe.

- Mindfulness
- Meditation
- Breathwork or breathing exercises
- Progressive muscle relaxation
- Grounding techniques
- Self-compassion exercises
- Emotional regulation exercises
- Mindful movement, like slow or restorative yoga or a gentle stretch
- Journaling (handwritten)
- Sensory exploration
- Dance
- Tai chi
- Qigong
- Somatic therapy

It can feel overwhelming to know where to start. If it's helpful, you can create a thirty-day plan for yourself. It doesn't need to be rigid, and if you start an activity and it doesn't feel right, you can always swap for another that might be more in line with where you are and what your body needs that day. Here is a sample plan for thirty days of exercise, grouped in a way that allows for you to build on previous skills and move from feeling disembodied to integrated embodiment.

Days 1 to 5: Build Mindful Awareness

DAY 1: MINDFUL BREATHING

Set a timer for five minutes and focus on your breath. Inhale through your nose, deeply and slowly, until you feel your lungs and belly fill up with air. Pause, and slowly exhale your breath. You might decide to focus on counting your breaths or creating a predictable rhythm with them, but you don't have to. If five minutes seems too long at first, you can adjust the time if that feels more comfortable. Don't worry about whatever thoughts might be crossing your mind; when you notice them, redirect your consciousness back to your breath. Notice the sensations in your body with every inhale and exhale without judgment.

DAY 2: BODY SCAN

Find a comfortable place to sit or lie down. Starting at the top of your head, scan each body part, top to bottom, front to back, side to side, or in any order that feels appropriate for you. Go slow and pause with each body part, taking notice of any sensations or tensions without judgment. If you feel tension anywhere, try directing breath into that part and exhaling to offer a release.

DAY 3: OBSERVE THE PRESENT MOMENT

Pick an activity that is part of your daily routine, that you normally do without giving it much thought (such as walking the dog, washing your hair, or brushing your teeth). As you're doing that activity, check in with each of your senses: sight, sound, smell, touch, and taste. What sensations do you notice? If you get distracted, that's OK. Bring yourself back to your senses to return to the practice.

DAY 4: FIVE SENSES CHECK-IN

Pick three to five moments throughout the day to engage each of your five senses. See if you can identify five things you can see, four things you can touch (or feel), three things you can hear, two things you can smell, and one thing you can taste. Observe this data without attaching a quality or judgment.

DAY 5: HANDWRITE GRATITUDE

Check in with yourself about three things you feel gratitude for today. Write them down one at a time, reflecting on any emotions or physical sensations present as you acknowledge each point of gratitude. Write down anything you observe within you.

Days 6 to 10: Developing Emotional Awareness

DAY 6: IDENTIFYING YOUR EMOTIONS

Notice five emotions you're feeling. You might want to download an emotions chart for guidance; there are many online to choose from if you need help sparking awareness. As you notice each feeling, become aware of any sensations or tensions you feel in your body associated with each emotion.

DAY 7: EMOTIONAL JOURNAL ENTRY

Either set a timer to write for five minutes or write at least one page of reflections on your feelings throughout the day. Describe how you felt for each emotion and what physical sensations aligned in your body. If you choose to do this in the morning, you might reflect on the previous day.

DAY 8: TAKE A MINDFUL WALK

Apply mindfulness to a walk. It doesn't have to be a rigorous walk; you can walk from the kitchen to the bathroom, to get your coffee, or from your car or public transport to your office, the gym, or to meet up with a friend. Take the time to feel each step you take. Notice how your body moves, how your weight is distributed. What part of your foot hits the ground first? Notice the sensations in your legs as you lift them and after you take a step.

DAY 9: EMOTIONAL BREATHING

Notice your emotions throughout the day. As you experience a shift in emotional intensity, pause and take three to five slow, deep breaths. Observe how this breath influences your emotional state. Are the feelings as intense? Did they shift?

DAY 10: LOVING KINDNESS MEDITATION

Imagine generating feelings of kindness and compassion for yourself and others. Visualize gathering these feelings and bestowing them on yourself and others. Notice what it feels like in your body to generate the feelings and receive them, as well as to generate the feelings and give them to someone else.

Days 11 to 15: Cultivating Embodiment

DAY 11: MINDFUL EATING

Choose one meal during the day to eat mindfully. With each bite, pay close attention to your five senses and notice the flavors, textures, smells, visual aesthetics, and tastes. Notice how your body responds to the different sensations and whether you have any emotional reactions.

DAY 12: GENTLE YOGA AND BODY SCAN

Make time for a short or long gentle yoga session today. Stay in the moment with each movement, noticing your breath and any sensations in your body without judgment. Honor any sensations that tell you to make adjustments for comfort.

DAY 13: NONSEXUAL TOUCH EXERCISE

Find a partner, romantic or platonic, for a nonsexual touch exchange. Check in with each other about any body parts you would like touched and any that are off-limits. Stick to your agreements and touch each other with varying kinds of touch and different intensity levels. Check in with every changed level of touch or intensity to see if it feels OK or should be stopped.

DAY 14: PROGRESSIVE MUSCLE RELAXATION EXERCISE

You can download a script from the internet or feel free to freestyle as you scan each part of your body. Tense a muscle group, hold it, and then release. Paradoxically, tensing the muscles helps to provide a counterbalance for deeper relaxation. Move through every muscle group, one by one, including the muscles in your face.

DAY 15: SYNCING MOVEMENT AND BREATH

Either with yoga, stretching, or a short exercise routine, sync your movements up with your breath. You might slow down your breathing. Give yourself time to notice the sensations in your body and check in with your breathing each time you inhale or exhale. Notice any tensions or a rhythm that feels good.

Days 16 to 20: Blending Mindfulness and Embodiment

DAY 16: LISTENING MINDFULLY

While in a conversation with someone else, focus on their movements as they speak. Notice your own physical and emotional reactions in response to their words.

DAY 17: ARTFUL EXPRESSION

Select an artful medium (colored pencils, paint, sculpture, charcoal, markers, and so on) and draw, paint, or sculpt what your emotions feel like. You can pick one emotion to explore in depth or include multiple emotions if you feel several in the moment. Don't use any words. Notice the sensations that arise in your body as you create.

DAY 18: EMBODIED SELF-COMPASSION

Look in the mirror and offer each part of your body kindness, compassion, and nonjudgment. Notice your emotional and physical sensations as you address each part of your body.

DAY 19: EMBODIED DANCE MEDITATION

Select a style of music or song that you like to move to. Don't worry about dancing well or using choreography. Just let your body move with the beats or sway of the song. Notice any physical sensations or emotions that arise. You can move as quickly or slowly as feels comfortable in your body and adjust to your level of physical ability.

DAY 20: MINDFUL COMMUNICATION WITH A PARTNER

Find someone to practice with, either a platonic or romantic partner. When in conversation, pause and take a moment to connect your breath, physical sensations, and emotions with each other. Track how you feel with each back and forth and make note of any stimuli that caused a bigger emotional reaction in you.

Days 21 to 25: Mindful Connection

DAY 21: CONNECT WITH NATURE

Spend some time in nature connecting with each of your five senses as you spend time in the elements. Notice how your senses register information in contrast to when you are inside. Notice any physical sensations and emotions.

DAY 22: EMBODIED SHOWER

When you get into the shower today, notice all of your five senses as the water hits your skin. What emotions and physical sensations are you aware of?

DAY 23: EMBODIED APPRECIATION

In front of the mirror, take time to practice gratitude for each part of your body. Notice the emotions and physical sensations that arise, especially as you move to your genitals.

DAY 24: GUIDED MEDITATION

Choose a guided meditation online or from another resource that emphasizes both mindfulness and embodied awareness. Notice your physical sensations and emotions with each breath without judgment.

DAY 25: MINDFUL MASSAGE

Pick a platonic or romantic partner for a nonsexual massage. Communicate to each other which part of your body you would like massaged (not breasts or genitals) and set a timer for five minutes each. Whether you are the massager or the recipient, notice the sensations in your body and your emotions as you give or receive the massage.

Days 26 to 30: Reflection, Integration, and Intention Setting

DAY 26: REFLECT AND JOURNAL

Reviewing the past twenty-five days, journal about how your relationship with your body and mindfulness practices have influenced your day-to-day life. Has it been easy to remain consistent? What has been challenging, if anything? What have you learned about your body and emotions, and how they are connected?

DAY 27: RELAXED BREATHING

Practice slowly drawing your breath into various parts of your body. As you inhale, target a part of your body to receive the breath. Hold your breath for a beat and slowly exhale. Notice the sensations in your body and any emotions that you may be feeling.

DAY 28: GUIDED VISUALIZATION

Find a guided visualization online (or perhaps you have one already) that facilitates the connection of your emotions and somatic sensations. Consider how visualization influences the feedback loop between your sensations or emotions. Does it allow you to be more present in your awareness of both?

DAY 29: EMBODIED MOVEMENT ROUTINE

Now that you've had twenty-eight days to curate more embodiment, what somatic exercises would you like to make a part of your routine? Create a routine to combine your breath and movement to further your capacity for grounding, somatic centering, and embodiment.

DAY 30: CREATE INTENTIONS

Draft a plan and set intentions for future embodiment practices. Which of these activities facilitated deeper integration for you? How might you apply some of these activities to your sexual practice of embodiment?

Embodiment is the cornerstone to pleasure, and pleasure is essential in returning to or amplifying desire. Practicing embodiment exercises may feel unsexy at times, but it is the development of heightened sensory awareness that can be a guide to having better sex, increasing arousal and your desire for more. It can also help to more readily build trust in your body for discernment around boundaries and limits.

Pleasure Points

- If you've been feeling numb, muted, or disconnected from your body for a while, it will take time, patience, and consistent practice to reconnect, but it is an important step in reestablishing embodied safety and the potential for pleasure.

- Talk therapy isn't enough to address trauma stored in the body. Embodiment practices can offer a path to a healing mind–body integration.

- Attuning to your body can help you develop emotional regulation skills, which can keep you in your window of tolerance and more present to experience pleasure and arousal.

Pleasure Reflections

- When you connect with various parts of your body, what emotions or physical sensations are you aware of? How do they impact your experience of pleasure?

- In what ways have you historically avoided uncomfortable feelings, and how might this play a part in your relationship with desire?

- What fears or barriers might keep you from fully engaging with your emotions or connecting with your body? How might you begin to work through these blocks? What skills, internal resources, or external supports might help?

How Do I Feel More Pleasure?

Unsurprisingly, one common reason for a drop in desire is that the sex you are having is not altogether that pleasurable. But pleasure is sometimes complicated, depending on how we've learned to prioritize it (or not). There are three parts to inviting more pleasure into your life: (1) removing obstacles to pleasure, (2) cultivating awareness of pleasurable moments, and (3) savoring the experience. Sounds easy, right? Well, it can be. And sometimes it can feel like a Sisyphean endeavor to carve out the time or permission for pockets of pleasure throughout the day.

Despite the prolific benefits of pleasure in our lives, many struggle to incorporate it with intention. Pleasure is intricately linked with positive emotions and happiness and is known to boost your mood and well-being through the release of endorphins and dopamine. A necessary component in reducing stress and promoting relaxation, the practice of experiencing nonsexual and sexual pleasure is a natural coping skill and protects your mental and physical health. Motivation, fulfillment, purpose, and a sense of meaning can be derivatives of pleasure, and they can serve as a buffer against anxiety and depression. Studies abound touting the benefits of pleasure on cognitive functioning, creativity, and longevity.[1] So, why can pleasure feel so elusive?

Isn't Pleasure a Privilege?

In a capitalist society, the relationship people have with pleasure can be complicated. When a system is too focused on profitability, the people who work and live in that system can internalize a warped view of themselves, in which their sense of worth or even morality is structured around their measured productivity. Pleasure can become detached from the experience of embodied enjoyment and can instead become a tally of achievement and validation.

Further, pleasure is promoted via consumer culture—keeping up with the Joneses, if you will—and it's encouraged by merging the idea of pleasure with competition, consumerism, and success. Economic inequality can exacerbate a drought of pleasure in a capitalist system, as those with less time and financial resources may find it challenging to prioritize savoring over surviving.

Additionally, values about pleasure (and productivity) are often shaped by cultural and religious positions, and may be difficult to reconcile as pleasure is seen in some religious or cultural contexts as a demarcation of poor character. Being told you are a bad person if you prioritize pleasure can frame it as an existential threat, evoking guilt or shame at the mere thought of seeking it out. Women often experience this kind of conditioning as they are taught to prioritize the well-being of others to their own detriment. An overdeveloped sense of responsibility for others keeps many people, women in particular, in a state of deprivation and rewards them with respectability should they adhere to the self-sacrificial script. As discussed in chapter 2, this is a great example of how identity can limit our willingness to pursue pleasure. If we fear losing social standing or safety by its pursuit, the desire for it can quickly be tamped down.

To avoid pleasure is to capitulate to a dehumanizing system, which requires labor and servitude without the expectation of reciprocity. As a result, centering your pleasure, both nonsexual and sexual, can be viewed as an act of empowerment and even activism; a reclaiming of somatic wisdom and enjoyment of the senses. Centering your pleasure is a declaration of your humanity and an assertion of the human right to well-being. Under systems of patriarchy, white supremacy, ableism, and capitalism (to name a few), only some people (rich white men) are afforded what is determined to be the *luxury* of pleasure. Why? Because *they've* earned it, they'll say, by virtue of who they are or how hard they've worked, as everyone struggles to establish balance in their lives to varying degrees. If everyone believed that pleasure was a right, there would be more demand for equality of it, and those at the top of the social hierarchy wouldn't be positioned with such disparity above the rest of humanity.

People with more power in any society may exercise greater agency in shaping their lives around pleasure, whereas those without the same time or resources may have limited access to define their own pleasure, let alone experience it. People in power often play a significant role in defining pleasure for those with less power, which can in turn influence how people with less power experience and seek it out.

There are also disparities when it comes to sexual pleasure. A study surveying over fifty-two thousand participants was conducted to look at the rates of orgasm among men and women* of all sexual

---

* The data are reported in gender binary terms and there is no information available about the rates of orgasm for people who identify as gender nonbinary, agender, gender nonconforming, or otherwise outside the gender binary.

orientations.[2] The study noted a 30 percent difference between straight men and straight women, coining it the orgasm gap. Such stark differences did not occur between men who have sex with men or women who have sex with women. But straight women came up last with a huge chasm of difference between them and the people with whom they're having sex. Disparities in pleasure equity are rooted in all kinds of patriarchal ideology, from the lack of consistent sex education to male entitlement and sexual double standards.

Pursuing pleasure is a commitment to autonomy in your body and a statement of personal power. It can fly in the face of systems that benefit from the exploitation of emotional and physical labor (at the expense of pleasure). Sexual pleasure is highly governed under patriarchal systems; women are often taught to experience their own sexual pleasure secondary to the pleasure of their partner, particularly if they are partnered with or having sex with men. On the other hand, women who have sex with or who are partnered with other women often experience their sexuality as something denied or fetishized within the framing of patriarchy. There is a double standard that male pleasure is a valid need and female sexual pleasure is a commodity to fulfill male pleasure.

In patriarchal societies, women and other marginalized gender groups have notoriously faced control over their bodies, aesthetic choices, gender expression, and sexuality. People in those groups who dare to experience pleasure on terms different than what is permitted within the narrow and self-serving mission of preserving power and pleasure for men are shamed. A noxious combination of shame and deprivation promises the rescue of a woman's character, but if she dares to center and prioritize her own pleasure, patriarchal thinking can render her immoral or unwell.

Pleasure does not need to be earned and it is not a limited resource to be doled out only to some people at the behest of others. It is an internal experience that everyone is inherently worthy of seeking out and experiencing. Balancing individual pleasure with social interests is a noteworthy task, and it could be argued that having pleasure as a resource can better equip you to be present for others. Pleasure, in and of itself, is not dangerous to the balance of humanity. Pleasure can counterbalance life's challenges. Feeling restored can make it easier to lend a helping hand to others in need. While I'm not suggesting a hedonistic plunge into pleasure that shirks any and all responsibilities in life, it is equally as destructive to yourself and others to live in a state of pleasure deprivation.

Am I Depriving Myself of Pleasure?

Factoring in the limitations on time and financial resources that many people face, it can be a challenge to determine how much of your relationship with pleasure is within your power to restore and how much is rooted in external factors. You may be someone who unconsciously lives in a state of pleasure deprivation due to internalized messages about worthiness that can be sourced back to the oppressive structures outlined earlier in this chapter, and there may be elements of trauma related to those structures that remain unresolved. Most people who live in a state of deprivation don't wake up and decide they are not deserving of pleasure, but they unconsciously structure their lives in a way that makes embodiment elusive. Pleasure becomes an idea for "later," after they've checked off enough items on a never-ending to-do list or are otherwise considered worthy.

Pleasure deprivation is largely tied to shame. Shame erodes a sense of worthiness and tricks us into a false sense of control—if we

can just *do* enough . . . perhaps then we'll *be* enough . . . and perhaps
then we can feel *OK*. Here are some ways a mindset of deprivation
can inch into everyday life.

- **Chronic Busyness:** Heavy workload, tight deadlines, time
  constraints, excessive chores, or feeling as if you constantly
  need to be doing something to be productive. It all can become
  so time-consuming that there is very little time for rest or
  pleasure.

- **Neglecting Self-Care:** Deprioritizing your needs for good
  sleep hygiene, balanced nutrition, regular exercise, and healthy
  boundaries make it difficult to have the energy for activities
  that bring you joy or pleasure.

- **Negative Thought Patterns:** This is not a bid for toxic
  positivity, but rather a reminder to check persuasive negative
  thoughts about yourself, others, or the world, as too much
  focus on the negative (while meant to be self-protective) can
  lead to a deprivation of positive experiences and moments.

- **Overcommitment:** Like chronic busyness, overcommitting
  yourself reflects difficulties with personal time boundaries and
  can be indicative of deprivation, given that it positions other
  people's needs and priorities above your own.

- **Unrealistic Expectations:** Pleasure does not have to be big
  or extravagant. Pleasure is often in the little moments and can
  be overlooked or deprioritized if it feels like an arduous task
  or another thing that requires lots of planning, preparation, or
  expense to do.

- **Too Much Technology:** Being overly tethered to your devices
  can be a sign of deprivation, as it can limit your connection to
  your body, to other creative pursuits, or to others in real life, in
  service of numbing out.

- **Perfectionism:** Perhaps the sneakiest tell of deprivation, perfectionism is the pursuit of safety through the elimination of vulnerability. A self-protective mind tells us that if something is (or we are) perfect, then worthiness is a guaranteed protection from shame or other consequences. But what perfectionism really does is keeps us in denial of reality (no one is perfect and even the definition of perfection is subjective and fleeting) and isolated from intimacy. Intimacy is about being fully seen, inclusive of our real and perceived imperfections. In fact, intimacy *requires* imperfection, and perfectionism is to deprive oneself of it.

It may still be difficult to discern if your relationship with pleasure is rooted in deprivation. This can come from the ability to detect external demands out of your control and ways in which you may be unconsciously setting yourself up for ongoing deprivation. Lacking pleasure in your life can take a toll on your well-being, so if you're feeling any of the following impacts, consider that it may be time to strike more of a pleasure balance.

- You constantly feel low, unmotivated, sad, or apathetic, or generally disinterested in things you used to enjoy.

- You feel chronically stressed out or exhausted with a level of chronic fatigue that does not relent even with adequate sleep.

- You have a hard time sitting still or relaxing, even when it's appropriate to be in a state of rest.

- You avoid social commitments or activities that invite pleasure or connection and instead spend your time alone.

- You have headaches, muscle tension, or other aches and pains, and you may have a change in appetite or sleep quality.

- You feel irritable or too easily frustrated, which can be a sign that you do not have enough pleasure or rest in your life and you are feeling resentful.

- You may struggle to find any inspiration or creativity, as pleasure helps to inspire and nurture new ideas.

CASE STUDY

Tara was busy, always so busy. She learned early in life that having a good work ethic made her more likable. And by likable, that meant she was someone who others could count on, even outside of work. She was the advice-giver, the mini-therapist, the built-in babysitter for all of her friends, but she didn't have anyone she could rely on. That didn't matter. Her coworkers, friends, and family counted on her, and that gave Tara a sense of purpose. Tara came into therapy because she was sure there was something wrong with her when she realized that not only had she stopped having orgasms during partnered sex, but she wasn't really interested in sex that much anymore. She didn't mind not having orgasms and she still wanted to have sex for her partner, as she wanted him to have the release he needed. If he was enjoying sex, that was enough for her, but she used to have more orgasms.

What changed? Some reflection on Tara's day-to-day life revealed that not only was she having less sex, and less pleasurable sex, but she didn't have any hobbies anymore and hadn't been on a real vacation in over five years. She'd been working hard for a promotion and was trying to show up for everyone else in her life. When I asked Tara who showed up for her, she got teary, and said, "I do, sometimes." Her desire to avoid being a burden and to ensure others were OK first had led to a pervasive pattern of self-deprivation. But now, Tara was terrified of changing how she showed up in the world, for fear that if she wasn't there for others, they would be angry with her, or she'd miss out on other opportunities at work. Asked what the last moment of intentional nonsexual pleasure she could remember was, Tara burst into tears. She couldn't remember anything in the past year or so. She made a commitment to change that with a daily pleasure practice, which didn't require massive changes in her commitments right away. Eventually, Tara was able to step back and seek more reciprocity in her relationships and more time to be in her body—and time for pleasure. Unsurprisingly, her orgasms returned after Tara made a commitment to herself to savor her sensory experiences of enjoyment.

If you're accustomed to deprivation, giving yourself permission to change is the first step in redefining your life and centering your own pleasure. Being intentional to stop thoughts advocating further deprivation from seeping into your mind can begin a shift toward changing your narrative and experience of pleasure. While affirmations are not a cure-all for the real-life concerns of poverty, racism, sexism, patriarchy, and so on, they can offer a momentary recalibration of your right to pleasure. Consider if any of these affirmations speak to you in a helpful manner, and/or consider writing some of your own to help you maintain a connection to pleasure, even on hard days.

- My humanity is enough to access pleasure in all areas of my life.

- My body is a source of pleasure and I have gratitude for my ability to feel its sensations.

- I celebrate the joy and pleasure of micro-moments and will look for pleasure in everyday things.

- I will prioritize self-care and rest to prime myself for pleasure.

- I release any guilt, shame, or feelings of worthlessness about experiencing pleasure.
- I will practice embodiment to tune into my sensations on a deeper level.
- I give myself permission to savor experiences of pleasure and not rush through them.
- I am open to receiving pleasure sexually and nonsexually.
- I am willing to explore new avenues of pleasure in my life.
- My pleasure is important and is my responsibility.

Building a daily pleasure practice is an integral way to cultivate opportunities for pleasure in your mind and body that can be sexual or nonsexual. Nonsexual pleasure, such as enjoying the texture of a soft blanket on your legs, is just as important as sexual pleasure, as it keeps the body primed and paying attention to things that feel good. Having a better developed sense of what feels good can amplify the sexual sensations that feel good, since you're already so practiced at holding space for your own pleasure.

Practice Pleasure Every Day

Dialed down to its most basic elements, pleasure is a sensory savoring. It's noticing sensations that feel good in your body and really taking note of your enjoyment. It's about slowing down long enough to notice, and then holding on a little longer to linger in the contentment of the sensations. In the book *Slow Pleasure*, Euphemia Russell introduced the world to the concept of microdosing pleasure,[3] which means inviting pleasure and savoring it in even the smallest of moments or most incremental ways.

Like any new practice, you might take some time to prepare by reflecting on the activities or experiences that you think could bring you pleasure—from the little things (like the smell of a fresh mandarin orange) to the big (like taking that trip overseas you've been dreaming of). Add to the list all of the activities, hobbies, or experiences you might enjoy or have enjoyed in the past, such as which books you'd like to read, which trails you'd like to hike, or what supplies you might need to start a new hobby. Prioritize your list based on your preferences and resources (time and financial), and make a schedule for tiny moments and a few activities here and there that may be more of a time commitment or cost.

Once you've got a plan, notice how you feel. What thoughts arise as you begin to step toward change? What do you notice in your body? As you begin to put into practice these opportunities for pleasure, keep your mindfulness practice alive, too. Notice the full experience with all of your senses in the present moment. Remember to stay open to new experiences and take pleasure in the experimentation of it all. Even if you try something that doesn't bring you pleasure directly, can you find pleasure in the seeking? Calibrate your goals so that they remain realistic, such as listening to one song you love each day or really savoring the taste of jam on your toast. Your pleasure practice can include moments of solo pleasure and pleasure with others socially— just being around people you care about can be pleasurable. It can be helpful to keep a gratitude journal to make note of the things and experiences you have enjoyed and how you felt emotionally and in your body during that pleasure. With that, you have something to reflect on as you adapt and evolve your pleasure practice and celebrate all the pleasure you're bringing into your life.

Sexual pleasure can build from nonsexual pleasure, as they are both sensory indulgences. Touch, taste, smell, sight, and sound can bring all kinds of pleasure to your body and mind, and they can ramp up your sexual delights. Creating erotic energy starts with creating an erotic environment. Consider the moods that turn you on and make pleasure accessible for you; build an ambient environment that is conducive, comfortable, and sensual. Be intentional with activities and accessories that heighten sensuality, like scented candles, music, lighting, and the texture of your sheets or furniture or undergarments. Exploring fantasies alone or with a partner can be pleasure-packed, especially if your fantasies are enhanced with other sensory play, like sensual massage or erotic audio, literature, or film, sparking conversation or playfulness. Create erotic rituals for yourself and/or with a partner to signify special moments and help transition from a mood state where pleasure is hard to access to one where pleasure feels more accessible.[4] Practice the art of flirting or teasing, or explore creating erotic art. The activities are limitless when the goal is mutuality and pleasure. Make note of whether you are *performing* eroticism and pleasure or *feeling* it. It can be tempting to fake it till you make it when you're building up a pleasure practice, but if it feels obligatory or hollow, you may be performing pleasure instead of creating or savoring it. Truly *feeling* pleasure often feels like a surrender; you may notice it and it may take some effort to get there, but you're not commanding it. It's something you relax into, receive, or enjoy.

Pleasure Points

- Inviting more pleasure involves removing obstacles, cultivating awareness and permission, and enjoying the sensory experience. Despite the many benefits of pleasure, it can pose a challenge to incorporate it if you feel you don't deserve it.

- Pleasure in a capitalist society is complex and heavily influenced by values around productivity. Economic disparities can deepen the struggle to prioritize pleasure over survival needs and separate it from competition and success.

- Culture and religion often shape ideas about morality and pleasure, and condition women to put others before themselves to their own detriment. This perpetuates social hierarchies by demanding women's unpaid emotional and domestic labor and limiting their pursuit of pleasure.

- Centering your own pleasure can be an act of empowerment, agency, and activism against oppressive and dehumanizing systems.

Pleasure Reflections

- How have gender norms, culture, and religion shaped your view, prioritization, and practice of pleasure?

- Consider the various power dynamics at play in your life. How do they shape your ability to define and access pleasure?

- Reflect on your day-to-day life. Might there be any ways you are depriving yourself of pleasure? If so, what variables contribute to this deprivation? How are you impacted?

- Is pleasure equitable in your relationships, especially around sex? If not, what factors have led to this disparity?

Chapter 17

How Do I Stay Connected to My Desire?

I invite you to take a moment to check in with your body. What do you notice, as you scan from the top of your head to the bottoms of your feet, from the front to the back, left to right? What sensations exist? What emotions might be connected to those sensations?

Checking in with yourself regularly is essential to keeping a strong connection and sustainable relationship with your desire. Desire, vitality, and pleasure can be spontaneous, but for the most part, are generated with intention. Staying connected to pleasure is a commitment to staying connected with yourself. You are not a light switch, you don't just turn on and off at a moment's notice. Instead, think about desire and vitality like seeds in a garden. Flowers rarely pop up in a garden unless it is tended to. Moving forward, this is your work: to invest in yourself, your body, mind, growth, relationships, and expansiveness. Are you ready to make the commitment to yourself and your pleasure? If not, what might you need to take care of first, to clear space for emotionally or logistically? Perhaps you have so much on your plate that the idea of adding one more thing to monitor feels overwhelming?

CASE STUDY

That was certainly the case for Aileen. She was tired of having a sexless life and tired of feeling disconnected from pleasure. A busy stay-at-home parent, Aileen craved some time for herself without the kids, without the family dog, and when she was really honest, without her husband, too. She was tapped out and tired of waiting for her husband to seduce her or take her on a date. She had asked many, many times, and outlined for him in detail how much it turned her on to be taken out for an evening (that she didn't have to plan). He kept saying he wanted the same thing, and so they were stuck in a sexual standoff of sorts. She was not attracted to his passivity, yet he wanted to feel desired, too.

Aileen was no longer willing to put her sex life to the side. Still frustrated with her husband, she decided to change her relationship with solo sex. At first she felt guilty. Shouldn't she be including her husband or initiating sex with him if she was feeling desire? After checking in with herself, she realized that she did not want to overfunction in their relationship anymore, and the idea of being the person to initiate sex and plan dinner dates brought up so much resentment for her, that she felt it was not the right time to loop him in. Instead, she focused on her own pleasure.

Aileen gave her husband notice that moving forward, he was responsible for the kids all afternoon one day out of every weekend and she needed him to take them out of the house completely. He balked and didn't want to agree. He was tired on the weekends, too. She held firm and told him to get childcare (out of the house) and find somewhere to go, because she needed three hours of quiet to herself and could not be responsible for how he parented in those few hours each week. She was terrified to hold this boundary and fearful he wouldn't follow through, so she made it clear that if he didn't, she'd go to a hotel for some downtime. Giving him that choice, he chose to take the kids to his parent's house for a while each week, to avoid the extra expense of a hotel.

With her protected time, Aileen invested in some new sex toys and a membership to an app for audio erotica. She created a ritual around getting undressed, tidying up her space, lighting some scented candles (she loved vanilla and musk) and massaging her skin with a fragrant body oil, while she took her time listening to erotic stories. After a few weeks of this practice, she began to feel sensations of arousal in her body and she decided to try out one of her new toys.

Committed to trying new things, she immersed herself in a nonsexual daily pleasure practice and within two months, she felt more energy, more contentment, and more overall joy in her life. Her husband noticed and was curious about the shift, feeling insecure, and wondered if she was having an affair. Aileen assured him she was not, but was not yet ready to share with him her recommitment to her own pleasure. It felt like something just for her and she was worried that if she shared with him what she was doing, he would try to get involved.

While Aileen yearned for him sexually, protecting this

solo practice was essential to her. It was the first time in her life she was so invested in her own pleasure, boundaries, and time. After another month, Aileen finally shared what she'd been up to with her husband. He was shocked! At first he was angry—how could she be taking so much time to herself to masturbate? He was personally quick about it, usually "getting it out of the way" in the shower each day. His anger subsided and he soon felt envious that Aileen was having so much pleasure without him. Didn't she want him?

After a long discussion one night, Aileen suggested that he develop his own pleasure practice and she offered to take the kids somewhere for a few hours every week. He declined at first, but then decided he would give it a try. He found that when he did get contemplative about his own pleasure, he missed Aileen's touch, desperately. When she later got home with the kids, he put on a movie for them and brought her into the bedroom where they made love for the first time in a year.

Staying Connected to Yourself

Committing to yourself, to your vitality, to your pleasure is a commitment to your relationship (if you're in one). Even if your partner isn't willing to do their own work at the same time you're doing yours, your shift will be felt. It may help you make some difficult decisions about the partnership or it can help you find a path to each other. It's not your partner's responsibility to revive your relationship with desire—it's yours. Doing the work might shake things up in your relationship and within yourself.

At the risk of sounding redundant, staying connected to your desire is as much about sexual moments as it is about developing or reviving an integrated theme of eroticism and sensuality in your day-to-day experience of yourself. What that means is up to you, but there are a few themes and steps that can help. Where to start depends on where you are and what you perceive to be the biggest obstacles in your relationship with pleasure and desire. Is it time? Then how will you reorganize your schedule to allow for even the tiniest moments of self-care, embodiment, and pleasure? Is it shame? Deconstructing shame can be tedious work, but if it is your biggest block, how might you start letting go? Is it the quality of your partnership? What are your needs and values, and how have you communicated them (with yourself and your partner)?

Personal reflection is the start of an ongoing journey of sexual empowerment, pleasure enhancement, and having the sex life you want. What is your movement practice? How can you find a few moments each day to recenter your awareness in your body and practice the art of embodied reflection? Perhaps keeping a journal to note the intimate thoughts and feelings you experience on this path can help you be more intentional and to serve as a point of reference for your growth. None of this is rocket science, but it does require your time and attention, which may be your most scarce resources. That lack of time and attention is a real dilemma and one that may not have an easy solution. The real growth is in your relationship with yourself, and that requires an investment and a willingness to be curious and authentic, no matter what you learn.

What has brought me back to my own eroticism was a shift in my self-care and erotic education. Even as a sex therapist, I learn new things about sex and pleasure every day and for me, that can be a source of dopamine and intrigue. Perhaps consider diving into a more intentional sex education of sorts. Take some online courses about anatomy, read other books about your body and sexuality, other peoples' desires and sexual experiences, or subscribe to your preferred medium of erotica. Reading other peoples' stories at first brought up a lot of frustration for me. I was jealous of the hot sex they were having. But holding space for that jealousy, without judging it, gave me room to enjoy what I was consuming. And then, I started sharing what I was reading, watching, and listening to with my partner, and it became a new launchpad for our erotic life together. It was easier to talk about other people having sex than it was to rehash what wasn't happening between us. This made our interactions around sex more playful and sparked new passion.

Staying Connected with a Partner

Speaking of partners, one of the most common questions I get from women is, "How do I talk to my partner about this?" This can be delicate, especially if you're partnered with someone who is more sensitive to criticism or rejection, has reacted with volatility or shut down when you broached the subject.

Approaching a conversation about how to improve your sex life can be easier when you lead with vulnerability and openness and frame your part of the conversation with "I" statements instead of "you" statements. Start the conversation at a time other than when you're having sex, and try to do so when you're both in a headspace where you can have the conversation constructively. When you're ready, here are a few tips to help the conversation along.

- Express your feelings in earnest.
- Share positive memories of your sex life together.
- Discuss some recurrent or new fantasies you've been having lately and ask them about their fantasies.

- Frame the conversation as mutual exploration, education, and relationship growth.
- Communicate your needs in the interest of connecting deeper.
- Discuss changes in your sexual preferences and how to make space for something new.
- Express a desire for variety or novelty, and gauge how important that is for your partner, too.
- Address challenges you've been feeling with connecting to your own pleasure.

If your partner is struggling with this conversation or with making changes to your sex life, remember to approach with compassion, curiosity, and nonjudgment. What challenges might they be dealing with? Practice active listening to hold space for their concerns without jumping into solution mode. Be patient as you may have a different pace in mind for reviving your sex life. Reassure your partner that you're bringing this to their attention because you want to become more intimate with them—if that's what you want. Or be honest about what you need if they are not part of that equation. Lastly, evaluate your expectations and bottom lines. If your partner is not willing to join you on this journey of sexual and emotional growth, you need space to grieve, and other decisions may need to be made. But you *can* affect change in your relationship just by working on yourself.

Staying Connected with Community

It might sound counterintuitive, but having a great sex life sometimes means connecting with other people who are also committed to having amazing sex, with or without you. What are your agreements with your friends about discussing sex? Do you have a friend or peer group that is dedicated to sex positivity? If so, great! Be intentional in your exploration together. Take classes or go to events together, such as workshops related to sexuality, kink, or sexual health. Look for sex-positive meetups, discussion groups, book clubs, panel discussions, or gatherings coordinated by sex-positive individuals or professionals. Conferences and expos can be a great way to meet many sex professionals, learn about new sexual research and see what is trending as it relates to new books and ideas. Take some erotic dance classes, like pole dancing or burlesque, or other forms of dancing that feel passionate to you.

If you can't find these activities near you, or cost is a barrier, consider starting your own book club or discussion group with friends or even in an online chat. Find some blogs or online forums and make it a social experience to immerse yourself in conversation with other like-minded people. One of the greatest barriers to pleasure is isolation. Change it up and connect with other people looking to alter their narrative as well.

If you want extra support or feel stuck in your exploration of pleasure, consider working with a sex-positive professional or a sex therapist. A professional can be especially helpful if you are facing ongoing shame, fear, or difficulties after implementing some of what you've read here, and if you want to address a history of trauma or if you don't know where to start.

The goal is to step into your agency. Identify what you want your sex life to look and feel like and claim it. Don't be passive, unless that is what turns you on.

You are empowered to take control and write your own narrative.

You're responsible for your own pleasure.

Great sex starts with you.

Pleasure Points

- Regularly scanning your body and noticing sensations and emotions without judgment can help you maintain a stronger connection with yourself and your desire.

- Staying connected to pleasure and desire often requires intentionality, especially if you've been disconnected from either or both for a while. This involves investing in yourself, your body, your mind, your play, your curiosity, and your expansiveness.

- Connect with others who are committed to having a great sex, even if you're not having sex with them. Engaging in sex-positive events, books clubs, discussions, or online forums can spark desire, help you stay close to people who are safe to learn with and foster a sex-positive mindset.

Pleasure Reflections

- What sensations and emotions do you notice when you check in with yourself after reading this chapter?

- What might be your biggest obstacle to pleasure and cultivating desire in your daily life? What ideas have you taken away from this book or other resources to devise a starting plan?

- What are you committed to in terms of setting intentions to shift your relationship with desire? How can you hold yourself accountable?

Conclusion

When I set out to write this book, I was deeply frustrated with the state of my sex life. One day, after not initiating sex for a while, my partner looked at me and asked, "Do you want to play later?" with a glint of boyishness and levity. That was the opposite of sexy *to me*, and instead of finding it arousing, it left me drier than a desert. We'd had this conversation before and I thought I had been clear that when this was his invitation to initiate sex, it had a cooling effect on any desire that might have been brewing for me. His approach felt immature. "I don't get it," he complained, "you want me to initiate sex, but when I do, you tell me it isn't working." That made me even more annoyed. In my opinion, it was a low-effort attempt that put the responsibility for creating an erotic experience back on me. I was burned-out. My desire was responsive and looking to be cultivated. So was his, and so we remained deadlocked in our dead bedroom. It was exhausting for us both to be so stuck and out of sync, and I was beginning to wonder if we'd ever find a path back to the erotic together. We'd discussed opening our relationship or inviting in other partners, but when it came time to take action, I had no interest in that, either. It was so baffling and uncharacteristic for me to be so disinterested in sex.

I wish I could tell you that my sex life flipped a switch, and everything was hot and erotic again, but it doesn't always work like that. Desire is like a garden; if you plant the seeds, water and nurture them, and pick the weeds, you'll likely see the efforts of your time blossom. But when a garden gets no sun, is ignored, or has incompatible soil, you won't find a noteworthy bloom in sight. My garden was a mess and needed a good sorting. I had to roll up my sleeves and examine where I'd gone wrong. One thing was certain—I'd been neglecting and ignoring my sexuality for a while. I was stuck in a cycle of avoidance, hoping the problem would resolve on its own and that one day I'd just feel sexy again and have desire for my partner. But passivity had not been a fruitful strategy, so it was time to get real with myself. What was going on with me? What was going on in my relationship? It turned out, a lot.

Only *I* could turn around my relationship with sex and that required a reckoning. I had to be willing to make changes and take responsibility for my own pleasure (or lack thereof). It wasn't just on my partner to bring erotic energy back into our relational space. I had to work at it, too. So why wasn't I? As much as I loved my partner, I'd stopped seeing him as a sexual being. Our relationship had gotten to a point where he was like a friend, roommate, or family member, not a lover. That was on both of us. Living and working together from home had us blending into the wallpaper—we stopped really seeing each other. Romance and sexuality had been replaced with logistics, Netflix binges, and conversations about whether the dog had pooped. Or whether we had pooped. Not sexy. There were other things simmering below the surface, too. I deeply resented my partner for operating on his own timeline when it came to addressing areas of our relationship that I felt warranted exploration and attention. I felt unmet and that his efforts to join me were taking too long. I was worried we were not going to make it and that thought was devastating. He was my person. But for a long time, it hadn't felt like it, sexually. Were we another couple sabotaged by the pandemic, who could work our way back into a relationship that felt aligned and lively? Or were our struggles insurmountable?

I didn't know, and the possibility that it was the latter had me feeling stuck and numb. My sexual disconnect was in large part a protection against the inevitable grief I knew I was facing. Inevitable? Yep. In addition to making lifestyle changes, like getting back into a regular embodiment practice, I was facing the reality that I either had to end this relationship and move on (which was heartbreaking to even consider) or stay, knowing that it didn't meet some of the needs that were most important to me in partnership. Facing reality was going to be a gut punch either way, so it was time to lean into whichever iteration of grief was ahead.

This dilemma wasn't the only variable responsible for my disconnect with desire. I had been neglecting my body, going through hormone imbalances from oral contraception and perimenopause, and working a lot. Like . . . a lot. So, how much of what I felt about my relationship actually had more to do with me and less with the quality of our dynamic? These are questions I am still working through. Therapists and sex therapists go through the same kinds of personal and relationship struggles that non-therapists do. We are all human; dynamic works in progress.

It's my hope that reading this book has given you a starting point to begin unpacking the layers of life that sit between you and desire. In no way is this book a light-switch remedy, because there is no sustainable bypass through the work. You might find a medication or an erotic catalyst here and there to jolt a surge of desire. But if there are more complicated impediments in your connection with yourself, with pleasure, or with a sexual or romantic partner, desire may feel chronically elusive. What fears come alive when you think about making changes?

When I looked at the changes I thought I needed to make, my biggest fear was that I would outgrow my partner, who was putting in the work, but not at a pace or direction that felt in line with my needs, growth, or own efforts. I feared that this relationship would no longer fit, and that in choosing myself, I'd have to say goodbye to a person I loved deeply. Speaking that truth to myself and to my partner was terrifying, but it allowed us to reimagine our relationship (once we got past the hurt and defensiveness). As much as I loved my partner, I was grieving big time—grieving the relationship I wanted, grieving the loss of my sex life, grieving my freedom. I got to a point where the grief subsided and I was ready to move on, with or without my partner. He had to be ready to step forward with me or I was going to step forward on my own. That was his work and I had been waiting to see if he would do it, all the while holding back on my own growth to avoid growing apart. Gratitude pours over me as I reflect on how we've grown together. But in truth, I was ready to leave the relationship in order to reconnect with myself and my desire. I didn't want to leave, but I was prepared to.

As an aside, not everyone has the choice to end a relationship so readily. Having the ability to leave is not a guarantee and for those of you reading who are unable or unwilling to leave your current situation, for whatever reason, there is still hope. Changing your relationship with desire is an inside job, and relational changes start with you. Waiting for your partner to change is passive and rarely leads to a successful relationship. Making changes within yourself can be the ripple you need within your relationship dynamic, which can make staying not only more tolerable but more enjoyable. Your relationship with sex is not for your partner, it's for you. You may have to decenter your partner's needs or limitations around pleasure in order to get back in touch with your own. Your pleasure is yours.

My relationship with desire changed when I stopped making it such a big deal and instead really listened to my body. Whenever I thought about having sex with my partner, it sounded nice in theory, and I wanted it mentally, but my body did not. I would push myself to initiate sex even when I felt apathetic or even repulsed—not because of my partner, but because of having to push myself to do another thing, a thing that I wanted to want but couldn't muster any enthusiasm for. I decided to stop trying and to start reevaluating my priorities. What was my body saying yes to, in lieu of sex? A few things came to mind immediately. Sleep was at the top of my list. Perimenopause had wrecked my ability to sleep through the night, and my energy levels were depleted. I was exhausted, and my body had nothing to give. Arousal was nonessential, so I had no energy for sex. I listened to my body and slept more, planning days on the couch and days when no one could contact me.

Several doctors had dismissed my claims that I was experiencing perimenopause. The rage that this experience made me feel (which is a symptom of perimenopause for some people) led me to a place of self-advocacy. I collected data through a daily hormone tracker and symptom log and found yet another new doctor. After I presented all the data, a provider finally offered me hormone replacement therapy. Adjusting to the treatment took some time, but eventually I was sleeping better and had more energy throughout the day.

But I still had no desire for partnered sex. Solo sex was available, and I gave myself permission to take the time to reacquaint myself with old fantasies. Surprisingly, they held less erotic charge than they once did. I was searching for new themes, images, and stories. It was thrilling! But when I thought about being sexual with my partner, still, I felt nothing. He was not initiating sex often, and I had stopped altogether by this point.

Still undecided about whether I wanted to remain in this relationship, I took a step back. My love for my partner never changed, but I felt called to tend to myself more. We agreed to be together when it suited us and to take space when we needed it in order to focus on our own goals and growth. Well, I needed a lot of space. He understood and gave it to me, which required a leap of faith for both of us. We accepted that perhaps these few years were just not going to be our most sexual years. Having known each other nearly twenty years, and after having dated for five years while enjoying incredible sex together for all but the last few, we knew our sexual potential—knowledge that at times amplified our sexual frustration and at times offered some hope that we'd get back to an erotically fulfilled life. Paradoxically, the decision to surrender to the powerlessness we felt in the face of our frustrations gave us more control. Stepping back into our foundation of friendship gave us space to redefine our romantic and sexual relationship.

It also gave me space to address other priorities, like finishing this book and getting back into the habit of exercising. I made a commitment to myself to prioritize the projects I was passionate about and to return to practicing daily movement. Prioritizing the nonsexual things in my life that felt meaningful reduced my stress and opened the room to be in relationship with my body and pleasure. Moving my body felt accessible, as it was no longer connected to an outcome. I just wanted to feel easy in my skin with gentle stretching, walking, and restorative yoga. Listening to my body gave me a path back to myself: back to my feelings—all of them, even the messy ones—and back to movement, which felt like freedom and, eventually, pleasure.

During this time, my partner and I talked a lot about our relationship, about what was working and what wasn't. We began to collaborate more effectively, focusing less on what we *should do* and more on how to *be* together. Taking this emotional space away from the problem of our sex life allowed us to enjoy each other's company differently. Eventually, we revisited the topic of sex, but this time without an agenda or a plan. Instead, we explored our fantasies out loud without fretting if one or both of us had no interest in entertaining them in the moment. Little by little, our resistance to being sexual together gave way to intimate touch and innuendo. This shift came from a place of want—not obligation or expectation. It had taken work and time, but finally, we both started to feel authentic desire again.

This journey can feel hard. Take your time. Listen to your body. Give yourself a lot of grace. You don't have to make any changes until you feel ready. Empowerment and resilience look different for everyone, so please do not compare yourself or your journey to that of anyone else. There is no right way to feel desire or to reclaim it, but my hope is that perhaps this book can help you make a shift that feels meaningful to you.

You are not broken.

Notes

1 Am I Broken?

1. Nagoski, Emily. *Come as You Are: The Surprising New Science That Will Transform Your Sex Life.* New York: Simon and Schuster, 2022.

2. Saini, Angela. *The Patriarchs: The Origins of Inequality.* Boston: Beacon Press, 2024.

3. Klein, Verena, and Terri D. Conley. "The Role of Gendered Entitlement in Understanding Inequality in the Bedroom." *Social Psychological and Personality Science* 13, no. 6 (2022): 1047–57.

2 Who Am I?

1. Hill Collins, Patricia, and Sirma Bilge. *Intersectionality.* 2nd ed. Medford, MA: Polity Press, 2020.

2. Appiah, Kwame Anthony. *The Lies That Bind: Rethinking Identity.* New York: Liveright Publishing Corporation, 2018.

3. Miller, Susan B. *Disgust: The Gatekeeper Emotion.* Milton Park, UK: Routledge, Taylor & Francis Group, 2004.

4. Valenti, Jessica. *He's a Stud, She's a Slut, and 49 Other Double Standards Every Woman Should Know.* Berkeley: Seal Press, 2008.

3 Why Can't I Get Over It?

1. Zoldbrod, Aline P. "Sexual Issues in Treating Trauma Survivors." *Current Sexual Health Reports* 7 (2015): 3–11.

2. Herman, Judith. *Trauma and Recovery: The Aftermath of Violence—From Domestic Abuse to Political Terror.* New York: Basic Books, 1997.

3. O'Loughlin, Julia I., and Lori A. Brotto. "Women's Sexual Desire, Trauma Exposure, and Posttraumatic Stress Disorder." *Journal of Traumatic Stress* 33, no. 3 (2020): 238–47.

4. Leavitt, Judith. *The Sexual Alarm System: Women's Unwanted Response to Sexual Intimacy and How to Overcome It.* Lanham, MD: Jason Aronson, 2012.

5. Betrayal Violence Institute. "Betrayal Violence Institute." Accessed [n.d.]. betrayalviolenceinstitute.com.

4 Am I Burned-Out?

1. Nagoski, Emily. *Come as You Are: The Surprising New Science that Will Transform Your Sex Life.* New York: Simon and Schuster, 2022.

2. Papaefstathiou, Efstathios, Aikaterini Apostolopoulou, Eirini Papaefstathiou, Kyriakos Moysidis, Konstantinos Hatzimouratidis, and Pavlos Sarafis. "The Impact of Burnout and Occupational Stress on Sexual Function in Both Male and Female Individuals: A Cross-Sectional Study." *International Journal of Impotence Research* 32, no. 5 (2019): 510–19.

3. Abramson, Ashley. "Burnout and Stress Are Everywhere." *Monitor on Psychology* 53, no. 1 (2022): 72.

4. ICD-11. "ICD-11 for Mortality and Morbidity Statistics—QD85 Burnout." World Health Organization, January 2024.

5. Papaefstathiou, Efstathios, Aikaterini Apostolopoulou, Eirini Papaefstathiou, Kyriakos Moysidis, Konstantinos Hatzimouratidis, and Pavlos Sarafis. "The Impact of Burnout and Occupational Stress on Sexual Function in Both Male and Female Individuals: A Cross-Sectional Study." *International Journal of Impotence Research* 32, no. 5 (2019): 510–19.

6. Silverstein, Shel. *The Giving Tree.* HarperCollins, 2014.

7. Montei, Amanda. *Touched Out: Motherhood, Misogyny, Consent, and Control.* Boston: Beacon Press, 2023.

8. Manne, Kate. *Down Girl: The Logic of Misogyny.* New York: Oxford University Press, 2017.

9. Nagoski, Emily, and Amelia Nagoski. *Burnout: The Secret to Unlocking the Stress Cycle.* New York: Ballantine Books, 2020.

10. Maté, Gabor. *When the Body Says No: Exploring the Stress-Disease Connection.* Hoboken, NJ: J. Wiley, 2011.

5 Am I Numb?

1. Rullo, Jordan E., Tierney Lorenz, Matthew J. Ziegelmann, Laura Meihofer, Debra Herbenick, and Stephanie S. Faubion. "Genital Vibration for Sexual Function and Enhancement: Best Practice Recommendations for Choosing and Safely Using a Vibrator." *Sexual and Relationship Therapy* 33, no. 3 (2018): 275–85.

2. Lembke, Anna. *Dopamine Nation: Finding Balance in the Age of Indulgence.* New York: Dutton, 2021.

3. Koob, George F., and Nora D. Volkow. "Neurocircuitry of Addiction." *Neuropsychopharmacology* 35 (2010): 217–38.

4. Yang, Jinyan, L. S. Merritt Millman, Anthony S. David, and Elaine C. M. Hunter. "The Prevalence of Depersonalization-Derealization Disorder: A Systematic Review." *Journal of Trauma & Dissociation* 24, no. 1 (2023): 8–41.

5. Mangiulli, Ivan, Henry Otgaar, Marko Jelicic, and Harald Merckelbach. "A Critical Review of Case Studies on Dissociative Amnesia." *Clinical Psychological Science* 10, no. 2 (2022): 191–211.

6. Shining, Phil, and Nicol Michelle Epple. *Exploring Sexuality and Spirituality: An Introduction to an Interdisciplinary Field.* Amsterdam: Brill Rodopi, 2021.

7. Thomtén, Johanna, and Steven J. Linton. "A Psychological View of Sexual Pain Among Women: Applying the Fear-Avoidance Model." *Women's Health* 9, no. 3 (2013): 251–63.
Fogel Mersy, Lauren, and Jennifer A. Vencill. *Desire: An Inclusive Guide to Navigating Libido Differences in Relationships.* Boston: Beacon Press, 2024.

8. Crosby, Courtney L., Patrick K. Durkee, Anna G. B. Sedlacek, and David M. Buss. "Mate Availability and Sexual Disgust." *Adaptive Human Behavior and Physiology* 7, no. 3 (2021): 261–80.
de Jong, Peter J., Mark van Overveld, and Charmaine Borg. "Giving in to Arousal or Staying Stuck in Disgust? Disgust-Based Mechanisms in Sex and Sexual Dysfunction." *Journal of Sex Research* 50, no. 3–4 (2013): 247–62.

6 Am I Angry or Bitter?

1. Stoller, K. Paul. *Oxytocin: The Hormone of Healing and Hope.* Santa Fe, NM: Dream Treader Press, 2012.

2. Rokach, Ami, and Sybil H. Chan. "Love and Infidelity: Causes and Consequences." *International Journal of Environmental Research and Public Health* 20, no. 5 (2023): 3904.

3. Chemaly, Soraya. *Rage Becomes Her: The Power of Women's Anger.* New York: Atria Paperback, 2018.

8 Do I Have to Say Yes?

1. Farida, D. *69 Positions to Lose Your Virginity.* Independently published, 2024.

2. National Sexual Violence Resource Center. "Statistics In-Depth." 2015. nsvrc.org/statistics/statistics-depth.

3. van Anders, Sari M., Debby Herbenick, Lori A. Brotto, Emily A. Harris, and Sara B. Chadwick. "The Heteronormativity Theory of Low Sexual Desire in Women Partnered with Men." *Archives of Sexual Behavior* 51, no. 1 (2022): 391–415.

4. Saini, Angela. *The Patriarchs: The Origins of Inequality.* Boston: Beacon Press, 2024.

9 Do I Feel Desired or Objectified?

1. van Anders, Sari M., Debby Herbenick, Lori A. Brotto, Emily A. Harris, and Sara B. Chadwick. "The Heteronormativity Theory of Low Sexual Desire in Women Partnered with Men." *Archives of Sexual Behavior* 51, no. 1 (2022): 391–415.

2. Martin, Wednesday. *Untrue: Why Nearly Everything We Believe About Women, Lust, and Infidelity Is Wrong and How the New Science Can Set Us Free.* New York: Little, Brown Spark, 2019.

3. If you'd like to read more about these subjects, I recommend *The Patriarchs: The Origins of Inequality* by Angela Saini, *The Right to Sex* by Amia Srinivasan, *Women Who Run with the Wolves* by Clarissa Pinkola Estés, and *Why Women Have Better Sex Under Socialism* by Kristen Ghodsee.

4. Nussbaum, Martha C. *Creating Capabilities: The Human Development Approach.* Hyderabad, India: Orient Blackswan, 2011.

5. Calogero, Rachel M., Stacey Tantleff-Dunn, and J. Kevin Thompson, eds. *Self-Objectification in Women: Causes, Consequences, and Counteractions.* American Psychological Association, 2011.

10 Are We Compatible?

1. Day, Lisa C., Amy Muise, Samantha Joel, and Emily A. Impett. "To Do It or Not to Do It? How Communally Motivated People Navigate Sexual Interdependence Dilemmas." *Personality and Social Psychology Bulletin* 41, no. 6 (2015): 791–804.

2. Wise, Nan. *Why Good Sex Matters: Understanding the Neuroscience of Pleasure for a Smarter, Happier, and More Purpose-Filled Life.* Boston: Houghton Mifflin Harcourt, 2020.

3. This data was sourced 12/30/23 from a Modern Intimacy survey, completed by a total of 153 participants.

4. Arenella, Katherine, Abby Girard, and Jennifer Connor. "Desire Discrepancy in Long-Term Relationships: A Qualitative Study with Diverse Couples." *Family Process* (2024).

5. Martin, Wednesday. *Untrue: Why Nearly Everything We Believe About Women, Lust, and Infidelity Is Wrong and How the New Science Can Set Us Free.* New York: Little, Brown Spark, 2019.

11 Am I a Partner or a Parent?

1. Fahs, Breanne, and Eric Swank. "The Other Third Shift?: Women's Emotion Work in Their Sexual Relationships." *Feminist Formations* 28, no. 3 (2016): 46–69.

2. Anderson, E. "Hermeneutic Labor: The Gendered Burden of Interpretation in Intimate Relationships Between Women and Men." *Hypatia* 38, no. 1 (2023): 177–97.

3. Wezerek, Gus, and Kristen R. Ghodsee. "Women's Unpaid Labor Is Worth $10,900,000,000,000." *The New York Times*, March 5, 2020.

4. Harris, Emily A., Aki M. Gormezano, and Sari M. van Anders. "Gender Inequities in Household Labor Predict Lower Sexual Desire in Women Partnered with Men." *Archives of Sexual Behavior* 51, no. 3 (2022): 3847–70.

5. Jeung, Da-Yee, Changsoo Kim, and Sei-Jin Chang. "Emotional Labor and Burnout: A Review of the Literature." *Yonsei Medical Journal* 59, no. 2 (2018): 187–93.

6. Guidi, Jenny, Marcella Lucente, Nicoletta Sonino, and Giovanni A. Fava. "Allostatic Load and Its Impact on Health: A Systematic Review." *Psychotherapy and Psychosomatics* 90, no. 1 (2020): 11–27.

7. Rodsky, Eve. *Fair Play: A Game-Changing Solution for When You Have Too Much to Do (and More Life to Live)*. New York: G. P. Putnam's Sons, 2021.

8. Tatkin, Stan. *We Do: Saying Yes to a Relationship of Depth, True Connection, and Enduring Love*. Louisville, CO: Sounds True, 2018.

12 Are We Even Attracted to Each Other?

1. Crenshaw, Theresa L. *The Alchemy of Love and Lust: How Sex Hormones Influence Our Relationships*. New York: Pocket Books, 1996.

2. Gentille, Francesca. *The Neurobiology of Love and Lust*. Compiled handout, 2022.

13 What Actually Turns Me On?

1. Saini, Angela. *The Patriarchs: The Origins of Inequality*. Boston: Beacon Press, 2024.

14 What Are My Needs, Boundaries, and Values?

1. Rosenberg, Marshall B. *Nonviolent Communication: A Language of Life: Life-Changing Tools for Healthy Relationships*. Encinitas, CA: Puddle Dancer Press, 2015.

16 How Do I Feel More Pleasure?

1. Laan, Ellen T. M., Verena Klein, Marlene A. Werner, Rik H. W. van Lunsen, and Erick Janssen. "In Pursuit of Pleasure: A Biopsychosocial Perspective on Sexual Pleasure and Gender." *International Journal of Sexual Health* 33, no. 4 (2021): 516–36.

2. Frederick, David A., H. Kate St. John, Justin R. Garcia, and Elisabeth A. Lloyd. "Differences in Orgasm Frequency Among Gay, Lesbian, Bisexual, and Heterosexual Men and Women in a U.S. National Sample." *Archives of Sexual Behavior* 47, no. 1 (2017): 273–88.

3. Russell, Euphemia. *Slow Pleasure: Explore Your Pleasure Spectrum*. Hardie Grant Books, 2022.

4. Nagoski, Emily. *Come Together: The Science (and Art!) of Creating Lasting Sexual Connections*. New York: Ballantine Books, 2024.

Acknowledgments

Thank you to Biren for five challenging and beautiful years. Ours has been a long journey, one filled with growth, healing, and so much love. Thank you for your support in writing this book and being willing to share parts of our process with the world.

Thank you to all the people I've worked with, who have entrusted me to help them on their quest toward a relationship with sex that is unburdened by dullness or limitation, fear or shame, exploitation or pain. Without your courage, this book would not have been possible.

Thank you to my team at Modern Intimacy for giving me grace during the process of writing this book, support when I felt unsure, and for your love of the work we do. Thank you especially to Kayla for helping me organize the research and references for this book.

Thank you to Batya Rosenblum, Sara Zatopek, and the rest of the team at The Experiment, not least Matthew Lore, Beth Bugler, Zach Pace, and Besse Lynch, for helping to bring this book to fruition. I so appreciate your patient edits and tireless assistance in helping me shape what was in my head into a meaningful book!

Index

About the Author

Dr. Kate Balestrieri is a licensed clinical and forensic psychologist and certified sex therapist focused on helping people heal from trauma and addiction, improve their relationships, and have better sex lives. She is the founder of Modern Intimacy, a counseling practice that operates across ten states and offers coaching internationally. Dr. Kate is a passionate advocate for sex positivity, mental health, relational health, and social justice. She works with individuals and couples, primarily around treating trauma and concerns that fall along the intersection of mental health, sexuality, and relationships.

modernintimacy.com | ⓘ drkatebalestrieri | ♪ drkatebalestrieri